PLAYING WITH

Lucy Sanctuary

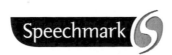
Speechmark

Published by

Speechmark Publishing Ltd, Sunningdale House, 43 Caldecotte Lake Drive,
Milton Keynes MK7 8LF, United Kingdom
Tel: +44 (0)1908 277177   Fax: +44 (0)1908 278297
www.speechmark.net

Designed by Moo Creative (Luton)

002-5792 - Printed in the United Kingdom by CMP (uk) Ltd

British Library Cataloguing in Publication Data
A catalogue record for this book is available from the British Library.

ISBN: 978 0 86388 915 8

CONTENTS

ACKNOWLEDGEMENTS

I would like to thank:

Jo Gilmore for her support and advice, for being an amazing speech and language therapist and an even more amazing friend;

Sarah Norman and Judy Avery for their encouragement and support;

Frances and Claire Burnham, Una Kroll and Tracey Fricker for putting up with me throughout the writing of this book;

Hilary and Stephanie for giving me this opportunity;

All the children who have played these games and enabled me to write this book.

This book is dedicated to my children, Phoebe and Felix Sanctuary.

INTRODUCTION

Why do some children need support to use speech sounds?

Children usually start saying single words by 12 months (Flynn & Lancaster, 1996). By four and a half years, most children can use nearly all of the 24 consonant speech sounds that are in the English language, for example, **m, b, p, s, k** (Grunwell, 1985). These speech sounds follow a developmental order: most children start saying the speech sounds **m, n, b, p, t, d, w** between 18 months and two years of age (Grunwell, 1985).

The development of speech sounds in children's talking

One and half years old to two years old	m, n, p, b, t, d, w
Two years old to two and a half years old	m, n, p, b, t, d, w Some children start saying h, k, g and ng (as in ing) These sounds are made at the back of the mouth.
Two and a half years old to three years old	m, n, p, b, t, d, w, h, k, g, ng, f, s, y Some children start to say l.
Three years old to three and a half years old	m, n, p, b, t, d, w, h, k, g, ng, f, s, y, l Some children start to say ch and sh.
Three and a half years old to four and a half years old	m, n, p, b, t, d, w, h, k, g, ng, f, s, z, y, l, sh, ch, j. Some children start to say r.

(Source: Grunwell, 1985)

However, not all children acquire the consonant speech sounds in the typical developmental order. For example, some children need help to say **k** and **g**, which are speech sounds made at the back of the mouth. They often use the earlier-developing speech sounds **t** and **d**, which are made at the front of the mouth, instead of **k** and **g**, in their talking.

There are various reasons why some children need support to use speech sounds. Listed below are some factors that can affect the development of speech sounds:

- Hearing impairments.

- Some children have frequent colds and ear infections such as glue ear, which can make it difficult for them to hear speech sounds accurately. We need to be able to hear a speech sound clearly in order to copy it and say it accurately. Difficulties hearing a speech sound can result in difficulties saying it.

- Attention and listening difficulties and short concentration spans can result in difficulties hearing speech sounds accurately. Children with these difficulties often miss important visual information about how we say speech sounds, for example the shape of our lips, where we put the tongue. This can affect the child's ability to say speech sounds correctly.

- Some children develop more slowly than others and need more time to use speech sounds (developmental delay).

- Children need to hear people talking in order to learn how to use speech sounds. Lack of opportunities to hear speech can affect the development of speech sounds.

- Using a dummy or sucking a bottle until two and a half or three can restrict the range of tongue movements a child makes, and this can affect their speech. For example, some children who use a dummy for a long time say the speech sounds **k** and **g**, which are made at the back of the mouth, instead of the speech sounds **t** and **d**, which are made at the front of the mouth. This is because the dummy restricts movement of the tongue tip, which we use to say the speech sounds **t** and **d**.

- Some children have difficulty co-ordinating the movements needed for speech, for example tongue movements, lip movements, breath support, because they have speech disorders or developmental verbal dyspraxia (DVD). Developmental verbal dyspraxia "is a condition where the child has difficulty in making and co-ordinating the precise movements which are used in the production of spoken language, although there is no damage to muscles or nerves" (Ripley *et al*, 1997). The child knows what they want to tell you, but difficulties co-ordinating the precise movements needed to say it, for example sequencing tongue movements and lip movements, can make it very hard for listeners to understand. In other words, what the child says does not match what they want to say: "My mouth won't co-operate with my brain" (quote from Kevin, aged 13 in Stackhouse, 1992).

- Speech sound difficulties are often found in families, so there might be other family members who have had help to say speech sounds accurately.

How does difficulty using speech sounds affect children?

Children with speech sound difficulties are often hard for people outside the family to understand. Children can become reluctant to talk as they are worried that others will not understand what they want to say. Speech sound difficulties can prevent a child from taking part in nursery and classroom activities and limit their ability to express themselves – to ask questions, to give opinions, to tell stories, etc. Children often worry that, if they put their hand up to answer a question, no one will understand what they say and other children might laugh at them. Communication difficulties can lead to low self-confidence and low self-esteem.

The speech sound p

You may like to know that:

- Most children start to say the speech sound **p** at around 18 months (Grunwell, 1985).

- We make the speech sound **p** at the front of our mouths, by putting our lips together. To say the speech sound **p**, put your lips together, keeping the air inside your mouth, then open them to release the air. It is like a small explosion. Say **pie** to feel the lip movement and the explosion of air. If you put your hand in front of your mouth when you say **pie** you can feel the air released. This can help children to say **p**.

- The speech sound **p** is a quiet sound, not a noisy speech sound like **b**.

- The speech sound **p** is a short sound, not a long speech sound like **s**.

- Children may say **b** instead of **p**, for example **bear** instead of **pear**.

- Helping children to say **p** might help them to say other quiet speech sounds such as **t** or **k** (Dodd, 2005).

About this book

What is it?

Playing with p is a resource for nursery practitioners, teachers, teaching assistants, carers, speech and language therapists, and speech and language therapy assistants to use in order to help children to say **p** in their talking. It contains activities, games and ideas to use with children aged from three years old to seven years old. It can also be used with older children who have learning difficulties. Each section contains simple, easy-to-follow instructions and practical tips to help you support the child you are working with. All the materials can be photocopied and instructions are given to help you make the resources for activities. There are progress forms in each section to help you and the child record progress. There are examples of session plans at the end to help you use the book. *Playing with p* aims to:

- give children opportunities to hear **p** in games, activities and jingles

- give children opportunities to practise saying **p** in games, activities and jingles

- provide a clear, easy-to-follow structure for activities

- provide tips to help you support children who have difficulties with certain activities

- be fun!

How long should sessions be?

Keep sessions short and carry them out regularly, perhaps 15 minutes five days a week. Be flexible. For example, if the child is not able to concentrate for 15 minutes, perhaps if they have attention and listening difficulties, make sessions shorter and gradually lengthen them as and when the child is ready. If the child can concentrate for longer, you can increase the length of sessions. Every child is different and this book allows you to tailor sessions to suit the individual. Take sessions in a quiet environment so that the child can focus on the work that you are doing and will not be distracted.

How to use the book

The first seven sections follow the typical acquisition of speech sounds by children:

- Section 1 contains exercises for the mouth (oro-motor exercises). It aims to help children learn about their mouths and practise movements that can help speech, for example rounding and spreading their lips.

- Section 2 aims to help children say the single speech sound **p**.

- Section 3 contains short words that begin with the speech sound **p**, for example **pie**, **pear**, **paw**.

- Section 4 aims to help children say longer words that begin with the speech sound **p**, such as **pan**, **park**, **pig**.

- Section 5 contains words that end with the speech sound **p**, such as **sheep**, **cup**, **hop**.

- Section 6 contains words that begin with **p** and have more than one syllable, such as **puppy**, **poppy**, **pelican**.

- Section 7 provides opportunities to use all the words presented in the book in phrases and sentences.

Each activity section contains both listening and speaking activities. This gives the child opportunities to hear the speech sound and see how to say it before copying it in a speaking activity. For example: round your lips or spread your lips, raise your tongue at the front of the mouth or at the back of the mouth.

Sections 3, 4, 5 and 6 include sets of jingles and rhymes which use the words you have been working on with the child. For example: "Would you like **pea pie** or **pear pie**? Mum wants **pear pie**."

At the end of each activity section you will find a progress sheet to help you and the child record the progress you are making in the sessions.

Section 7 contains activities that can be used with the words from Sections 2, 3, 4, 5 and 6 to enable the child to say words in sentences.

Section 8 contains ideas for games that can be played using the words from Sections 2,

3, 4, 5 and 6. These provide the child with more opportunities to hear the words you are working on and to practise saying them. Instructions are given for each game. Templates for resources are included with instructions on how to make them.

There are examples of session plans in Session 9 to help you use the book.

This book allows you to be flexible and to follow the needs of the child that you are helping. The amount of time you work on each section will depend on the child and the speed of their progress. There are ideas for making the activities more challenging and tips on how to make them easier so that you can tailor what you are doing to suit each individual child.

You will see that Sections 3, 4, 5 and 6 contain some of the same activities, for example 'Listen and guess', 'What's the word?', but using different words. The activities use different words in different sections – short words in Section 3 (e.g. **pie**, **paw**, **pea**), longer words that begin with **p** in Section 4 (e.g. **pipe**, **pot**, **pig**), words that end with **p** in Section 5 (e.g. **mop**, **tap**, **sheep**) and words that begin with **p** and have more than one syllable in Section 6 (e.g. **pizza**, **puddle**, **pocket**). The activities have been printed in full in each section for the following reasons:

- All activities can be photocopied and used alone.

- You do not have to refer back to earlier sections in the book in order to find instructions for activities, although the tips in Section 3 will be helpful in later activities too.

- You can access the book easily at any level. For example, if the child you are working with is having difficulty saying p at the end of words, you can start working on Section 5 without having to look back to earlier sections for instructions.

Tip

Photocopy pictures and resources on to card or laminate them for all activities so that you can use them again. Cut out the small pictures of the words you are working on to use in activities and games.

How to help the child to use the speech sound in their everyday talking

Changing the way a child speaks can take time. This can be very frustrating for carers and the child. Using one speech sound instead of another, for example saying **b** in words instead of **p**, can become a habit. In order to change this habit, children need regular opportunities to hear the speech sound they are not yet using and to practise saying it.

Children can often use the speech sound they are working on, **p** in this case, in sessions with support from, say, a speech therapist or a teaching assistant. However, outside the sessions they often continue to have difficulty using the speech sound in their talking. This can be demotivating for carers who are working with the child and for the child.

Change does not happen overnight and progress can be slow. This is perfectly normal and does not mean the child will never be able to change their talking.

Using progress sheets will help you and the child to see progress. Tell older children that it will take time to help them say **p** in their talking and that you will need to work on saying **p** regularly. Photocopy exercises and activities from the book and give them to carers so that they can work with the child at home.

Tips

- Be careful not to overload the child as this can be demotivating! Keep sessions short and fun so that the child remains engaged and interested. Give lots of praise and positive feedback to encourage the child.

- Avoid correcting the child as this can make them feel bad about their talking and it does not help them to change the speech sounds they are using. Instead of correcting the child, repeat what they have said *without the speech sound error* so that the child has an opportunity to hear the word that they want to say but cannot yet say in their talking. For example: if the child says "Can we go to the **bark**?" you say "Can you go to the **park**? You want to go to the **park**?" It can help the child if you repeat the word a few times in as natural a context as you can. For example: "Can you go to the **park**? You want to go to the **park**? We haven't been to the **park** for ages, have we? Which **park** do you want to go to?" (four repetitions of park). This can feel unnatural and be difficult to do, but it is worth trying!

- The jingles and rhymes at the end of sections give the child more opportunities to hear the words that you are working on. If possible, try reading them at set times, such as at bedtime, after dinner. As the jingles become more familiar and the child makes progress with their talking, start leaving pauses for them to complete the jingles. For example: "Would you like pea pie or pear _____ (**pie**)?" (See instructions for using jingles at the end of Section 3, p.60.)

- Encourage children to think about their talking so that they are actively involved in the speech therapy work. Give them information about speech sounds to help them monitor their talking. For example: "You said **bark**. **b** is a noisy speech sound. Listen: **b**. **Bark**. I said **park**. **p** is a quiet speech sound. Listen: **p**. **Park**" This can help children to listen and learn more about the speech sound they actually say and the speech sounds they want to say. Often children do not know that they are saying, for example, **b** instead of **p** in words. They need your help and support to realise that what they are saying is not what they want to say. Always model a speech sound or word for children so that they can hear it before they try to say it. Help older children to reflect on what they say. For example: "I said **park**. You said **bark**. Are they the same? Listen: **Park**. **Bark**." Raise their awareness by offering them choices. For example: "Is it **park** [hold out a fist as you say **park**] or is it **bark** [hold out the other fist]?" If the child cannot yet say **p** in words, they can choose between **bark** and **park** by touching one of your fists, either the fist that you held out when you said **bark**, or the fist that you held out when you said **park**.

How to use this book in the nursery or the classroom

- Play group or class listening games at carpet time – after registration, before break times, after lunch. You could put one of the resources to help children say **p** on the board, for example "Put a pea on a plate and say p" from Section 2. Choose a child to come to the board. Ask the child to listen and when they hear you say **p**, put a pea on a plate. Count silently to at least four before you say **p** so that the child has to wait. When the child has finished their go, ask them to choose another child to come to the board to listen and put a pea on a plate when they hear **p**. Let the first child say **p** for the second child. The children take it in turns to choose the next child to be the listener and to say **p** in the activity (see listening activities in Section 2, p.32).

- See instructions for games using words containing the speech sound **p** in Section 8, for example Charades. Play these with the group or class perhaps before lunch or at the end of the day before home time.

- Choose a word of the week from the words you have been working on. Put it on the board and tell the group or class that they have to clap or stand up every time they hear you say the word.

- Get a feely bag. Instead of pictures of the words you have been working on, find objects, such as pretend food (peas, pear, pie), a pan, a toy pig. Put one in the bag. Look in the bag and describe the object to the children. For example: 'It's an animal. It lives on a farm. It has got a curly tail and it grunts. Oink, oink. Hands up if you know what it is!' Put one object in the bag. Pass it to a child. The child feels the object through the bag, without looking, and guesses what it is. Change the object and give the bag to the next child.

- Read at least one jingle from the jingle sections in this book to the group or class. See instructions on ideas for using the jingles at the end of Section 3, p.60.

- Have a jingle of the week and teach the children actions to go with it to make the jingle more memorable and fun!

- Make your own jingles in class using curriculum vocabulary words that contain **p**.

- Start a **p** poster in the class. When you work on curriculum topic vocabulary such as mini beasts, habitats, our environment, put words that contain **p** on the poster (with pictures if possible to make them more visual).

- Play mouth exercise games with the group or class at carpet time or before literacy sessions. See Section 1 of this book for activities, games and pictures.

Tip

- Photocopy resources and give them to carers so that they can work with the child at home.

SECTION 1
EXERCISES FOR THE MOUTH

Section 1: Exercises for the mouth

Aim

To learn about our mouths and practise movements that can help speech.

How?

By giving the child opportunities to see you carry out the exercises and to copy them.

Resources

- A mirror so that the child can watch herself copying the exercises.

- Large pictures of mouth exercises (pp. 17–25).

- At least two sets of small pictures of mouth exercises with shapes on the back and at least two sets of small pictures without shapes on the back. Photocopy the sheet of shapes (p. 26) on to the back of a set of small pictures (p. 15).

- A dice.

- Template for a dice with a different shape on each face (p. 27).

- A set of the resource that tells you how to speak, e.g. *say it in a quiet voice, say it in a loud voice, say it in a sad voice* (p.185).

Instructions

1. Put the mirror in front of the child so that you both can see yourselves. Tell the child that you are going to do some exercises for your mouth! Before you start, ask her, for example, to show you her tongue, show you her teeth; open his mouth wide, give you a big smile. Encourage her to look in the mirror when she does these warm-up movements.

2. Look at the pictures, read the instruction and demonstrate the movement for the child using the mirror. Then say "You try!"

NB: the instruction to "smile like a granny" means to smile without showing your teeth (spread your lips).

Keep this activity short and fun.

Variations

When the child is familiar with the exercises, make them more challenging:

- Carry out the instructions to do a sequence of movements (pp. 22–25), e.g. *Can you put your tongue up to your nose and then down to your chin?* Always demonstrate movements for the child before she has a turn so that she can see what you want her to do.

- Take it in turns to roll the dice and carry out the sequence of movements that number of times. For example, if the child throws a 4, she has to move her tongue up and down four times.

- Turn the small pictures face down on the table so that you can see the shapes on the back but not the pictures of the mouth movement. Use the template to make a dice with shapes on the faces. Take it in turns to throw the shape dice at least twice. Turn over the pictures that have those shapes on the back. If you throw a circle, turn over the picture that has a circle on it so that you can see the picture of the mouth movement, e.g. *smile like a granny*. If you throw a star, turn over the picture that has a star on it so that you can see the picture of the mouth movement, e.g. *say ee*. Then throw the dice to see how many times you have to do the mouth movements. For example: if you throw a 6, you have to *smile like a granny* and then *say ee* six times.

- Put at least two sets of the small pictures (without the shapes on the back) face down in front of the child. Take it in turns to turn over two pictures and do the movement on each picture. If the two pictures are the same, for example, *blow a kiss* and *blow a kiss*, keep them as a pair. The winner is the person who has the most pairs.

- Photocopy the resource that tells you how to speak, e.g. *say it in a quiet voice*, *say it in a happy voice*, and cut it into cards. Put them in a pile, face down. Put at least two sets of the small pictures of *say ah, say oo and say ee* face down in front of the child. Take it in turns to turn a picture over, e.g. *say oo*, and take a card from the other pile, e.g. *say it in a loud voice*. Carry out the instructions. For example, if one picture is *say oo* and the other is *say it in a loud voice*, you have to say the speech sound **oo** loudly!.

- Place a barrier between you and the child so that you cannot see each other's pictures. Make sure that you both have at least two sets of the small pictures of mouth movements. Choose at least four pictures from your set. For example: *smile like a granny*, *blow a kiss*, *say oo*, *say ee*. Do not show the child. Arrange the pictures behind the barrier so that she cannot see them. The child watches you copy the mouth movements on the picture you have put behind the barrier and puts the matching pictures from her set behind the barrier. When she has finished, ask her to show you the mouth movements that are on the pictures she has chosen so that she has a turn at copying the movements. Then remove the barrier to see if she has the same pictures as you. When the child is familiar with this activity, reverse it so that she chooses the pictures and demonstrates them for you.

Tips

To practise lip movements:

- Try blowing whistles, blowing kisses, blowing bubbles, blowing musical instruments, whistling!

- Put on lipstick and kiss paper – one for the girls!

- Fill cheeks with air and then pop!

To practise tongue movements:

- Try holding a small food item, e.g. a Cheerio or a Polo on the skin just behind the top teeth (alveolar ridge). Tell the child to push against it as hard as she can with her tongue.

- Gently touch around the child's mouth, e.g. his chin, one of his cheeks, his nose. The child has to move her tongue to the place you touched.

- Put your tongue inside your cheek and push against the cheek! Try pushing back against the child's tongue so that she has to push harder.

My progress

Date	I can ...	☺/☹	I need to work on ...
	Do all of the mouth exercises without any help.		
	Do all of the mouth exercises with some help.		
	Do most of the mouth exercises without any help.		
	Do most of the mouth exercises with some help.		
	Do some of the mouth exercises without any help.		
	Do some of the mouth exercises with some help.		
	Do a few of the mouth exercises without any help.		
	Do a few of the mouth exercises with some help.		

Tips

Start sessions with a few mouth exercises, even when the child can do all the mouth exercises without any help. The exercises can be used as a warm-up activity before you start working with speech sounds.

say ah

say ee

smile like a granny

say ah

blow a kiss

say oo

15

move your tongue to the left

move your tongue to the right

move your tongue down

move your tongue up

can you

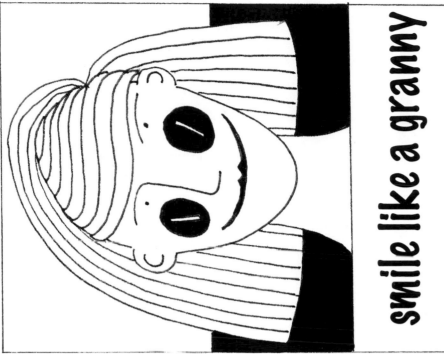

smile like a granny

and
then

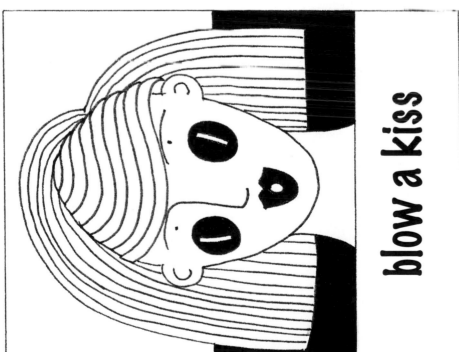

blow a kiss

can you

say ah

and then

say ee

can you

say oo

and then

smile like a granny

can you

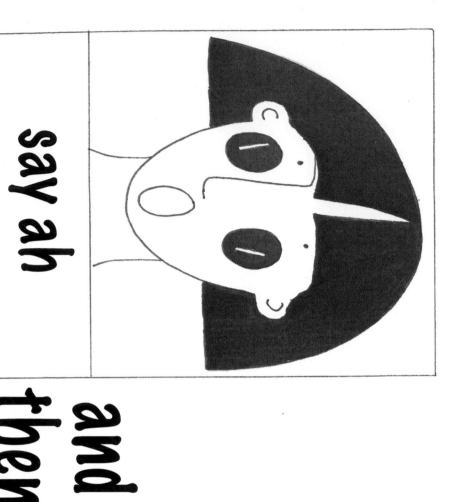

say ah

and then smile like a granny

can you

say ah

and
then

say oo

up to your nose

and
then

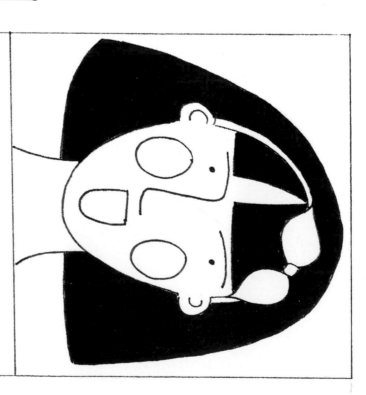

down to your chin

can you put your tongue

right

and then

left

say ah

and then

say oo

can you

24

can you move your tongue

side

to

side

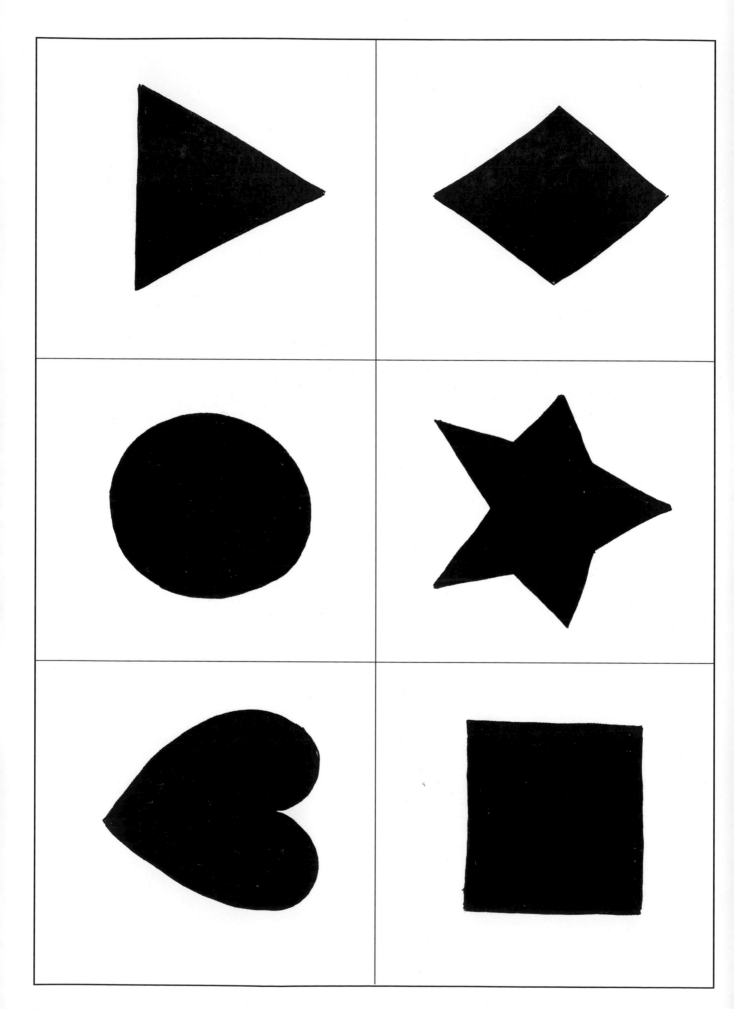

Template for a dice

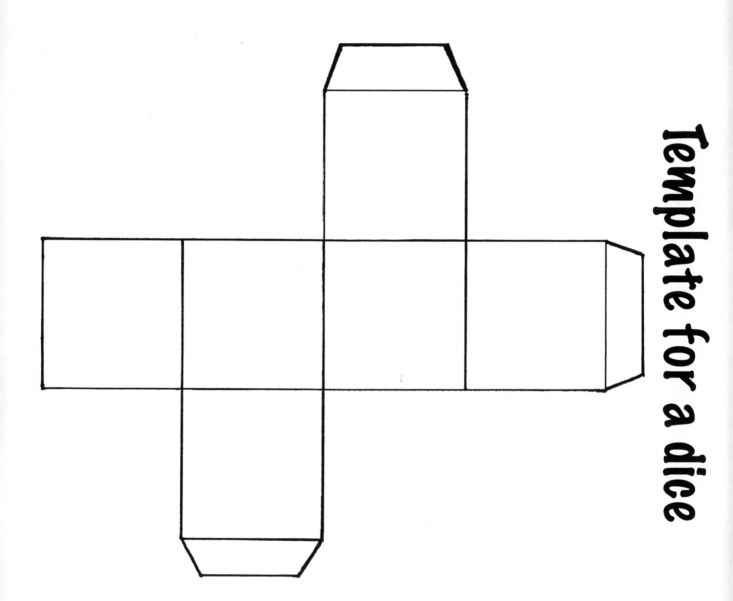

Template for a dice

SECTION 2

SAYING P

Section 2: Saying p

Saying the speech sound p (1) (Listening and speaking activity)

Aim

To say the speech sound **p**.

How?

By giving the child opportunities to hear, and see, you say **p** and to copy you.

Resources

- Picture of plates and cutlery and nine peas (p. 36). Photocopy the page twice. Laminate one page and put small pieces of Velcro or Blu-Tack on each of the peas, and three small pieces of Velcro or Blu-Tack on each plate. Cut out the line of peas from the other page and laminate it. Cut the peas out and put a small piece of Velcro on the back of each pea. Stick each pea on top of a pea on the picture of peas, plates and knives and forks.

- Picture of nine pigs and a pig pen (p. 37). Photocopy the page twice. Laminate one page and put small pieces of Velcro or Blu-Tak on each of the pigs, and nine small pieces of Velcro or Blu-Tak in different parts of the pig pen. Cut out the line of pigs from the other page and laminate it. Cut the pigs out and put a small piece of Velcro on the back of each pig. Stick each pig on top of a pig in the picture of pigs and a pig pen.

- Pictures of nine Pauls and a park (p. 38). Photocopy the page twice. Laminate one page and put small pieces of Velcro or Blu-Tack on each of the Pauls, and nine small pieces of Velcro or Blu-Tack in different parts of the park. Cut out the line of Pauls from the other page and laminate it. Cut the Pauls out and put a small piece of Velcro on the back of each Paul. Stick each Paul on top of a Paul on the picture of Pauls and a park.

Instructions

1. Read the instruction at the top of the page to the child, e.g. "Put a pea on a plate and say **p**." Before you carry out the instruction, say: "My turn!" so that the child knows you are going to do the task first. Then take a pea, stick it on a plate and say "**p**".

2. When you have finished your go, say: "Your turn!" so that the child knows it is his go. The child takes a pea, puts it on a plate and says **p**. Take turns until all the peas are on the plates, pigs are in the pen or Pauls are in the park.

Variations

Listening activities

- Tell the child to listen carefully and, for example, put a pea on a plate when you say **p**. Count silently to at least four and then say **p**. When the child hears you say **p**, he takes a pea and puts it on a plate. If the child finds this activity hard, demonstrate it on a toy or a puppet. For example: tell the toy/puppet to listen and put a pea on a plate when you say **p**. This gives the child an opportunity to watch the activity before he has a go. It also helps to reduce any feelings of anxiety he might have about taking part in the activity.

- To make this listening activity harder, again ask the child to listen carefully and put a pea on a plate when you say **p** but this time say at least four other speech sounds before you say **p**. For example: m s k sh **p**. Leave pauses between each speech sound to help the child listen for **p**.

- Try reversing the activity so that the child asks you, or the puppet/toy, to listen and put a cat on a cushion when he/she says **p**.

Speaking activities

- See how many times in a minute the child can put a pea on a plate, pig in pen or Paul in the park and say **p** in a minute. Use a one-minute salt timer to time him.

Saying the speech sound p (2) (Listening and speaking activity)

Aim

To say the speech sound **p**.

How?

By giving the child opportunities to hear, and see, you say **p** and to copy you.

Resources

- Template for a speech sound dice (p. 39)
- Hand prints to photocopy (p. 40).
- Heads, without hair, to photocopy (p. 41).
- Aliens to photocopy (p. 42).
- Coloured pencils/pens.

Instructions

1. Make a dice using the template. If the child cannot say any of the speech sounds on

the template (**m, n, w, d, t, h**) use the blank template for a dice (p.28) and write speech sounds that the child can say on it. For instance you could put three speech sounds instead of six, e.g. **m, m, n, n, t, t**.

2. Choose a template to photocopy for the activity, e.g. colouring rings on fingers, drawing hair on a head. Photocopy the sheet.

3. Roll the dice to choose a speech sound, e.g. **m**.

4. Choose two colour pencils, e.g. orange and blue. Say the speech sound **p** and draw a strand of hair on one of the heads. Change colour pencils, say the speech sound that you rolled on the dice, e.g. **m**, and draw a second strand of hair on the head. Repeat this ten times so that you draw five orange hairs and say **p** five times, and draw five blue hairs and say **m** five times.

5. Take turns to say the two speech sounds and draw a hair on the head (or colour in a ring, or draw an eye on the alien).

Variations

- Use the activity as a listening game, e.g. "When I say **p**, colour in a ring."

- Use the activity to practise saying **p**. For example, take it in turns to say **p** and colour a ring.

- Say **p** and draw a strand of hair on a head, change colours and say the speech sound you rolled on the dice, e.g. **m**, and draw another strand of hair. The child then says **p** and draws a strand of hair on the same head, changes colours and says the speech sound you rolled on the dice, e.g. **m**, and draws another strand of hair. Take it in turns until you have drawn at least twelve strands of hair on the head and said the speech sounds six times each.

- Take it in turns to say the two speech sounds, e.g. **p** and **m**, six times drawing strands of hair on the head after you have said each one. When you and the child have both had a go, there should be twelve strands of hair on the head.

Tips

*Help! The child says **b** instead of **p**! What can you do?*
- Try whispering **p** or saying **p** in a quiet voice.

- Try giving the child more information about the speech sound **p**. For example: 'You said **b**. That's a loud sound. Listen: **b**. I said **p**. That's a quiet sound. Listen: **p**. Remember, it's a quiet sound. Say it softly.'

- Take turns to do the activities with a puppet or a toy, i.e. you take a turn and then the toy has a go. This gives the child more chances to hear the sound and it takes pressure off him as he is not expected to speak.

My progress

Date	I can ...	☺/☹	I need to work on ...
	Listen carefully and put a pea on a plate when I hear **p** without any help.		
	Listen carefully and put a pea on a plate when I hear **p** with help.		
	Listen carefully to different speech sounds, e.g. **m**, **s**, **k**, **sh**, **p**, and put a pea on a plate when I hear **p** without any help.		
	Listen carefully to different speech sounds, e.g. **m**, **s**, **k**, **sh**, **p**, and put a pea on a plate when I hear **p** with help.		
	Say **p** without any help.		
	Say **p** with help.		
	Say **p** with other speech sounds, e.g. I can say **m**, **p**, **m**, **p**, **m**, **p**, **m**, **p** without any help.		
	Say **p** with other speech sounds, e.g. I can say **m**, **p**, **m**, **p**, **m**, **p**, **m**, **p** with help.		

What's the next step?

- I can listen carefully and put a pea on a plate when I hear **p** without any help. I can listen carefully to different speech sounds, e.g. **m**, **s**, **k**, **sh**, **p**, and put a pea on a plate when I hear **p** without any help. **Start listening activities in Section 3.**

- I can listen carefully and put a pea on a plate when I hear **p** with help. I can listen carefully to different speech sounds, e.g. **m**, **s**, **k**, **sh**, **p**, and put a pea on a plate when I hear **p** with help. **Carry on playing listening games from Section 2, but start to gradually include listening games from Section 3.**

- I can say **p** without any help. I can say **p** with other speech sounds, e.g. I can say **m**, **p**, **m**, **p**, **m**, **p**, **m**, **p** without any help. **Start Section 3.**

- I can say **p** with help. I can say **p** with other speech sounds, e.g. I can say **m, p, m, p, m, p, m, p** with help. **Carry on working on activities in Section 2 to practise saying p and doing mouth exercises from Section 1.**

When the child can say p at least 70 per cent of the time, gradually introduce activities from Section 3.

Tip

- To work out if the child can say **p** at least 70 per cent of the time, listen to him saying **p** ten times, e.g. saying **p** and colouring in a ring ten times, or saying **p** and drawing an eye on an alien ten times. If he says **p** correctly seven out of ten times, he has said **p** 70 per cent of the time.

Put a pea on a plate and say p

36

Put a pig in the pen and say p

Put Paul in the park and say p

Template for a dice

Say p and colour in a ring

Say p and draw a strand of hair on a head

Say p and draw an eye on the alien

SAYING P AT THE BEGINNING OF SHORT WORDS

Section 3: Saying p at the beginning of short words

What's the picture? (Speaking activity)

Aim

To say short words that begin with the speech sound **p**: **pie**, **pear**, **paw**, **pow!**, **pier**, **pea**.

How?

By giving the child opportunities to hear, and see, you say short words that begin with **p** and to practise saying the words.

Resources

- Large pictures of short words that begin with **p.** (p. 54–56).

- Small pictures of short words that begin with **p.** (p. 57).

- Page of two doors with question marks on each one and the instruction *What's the picture?* (p. 59). You will need to photocopy this page and cut along three sides of the doors so that you can open them to reveal a picture.

Instructions

1. Put the page with the doors on top of large pictures of words that begin with **p**, e.g. **pie** and **pear**.

2. Read the instruction at the top of the page to the child: *What's the picture? Open the door and see.* Before you open the door to see what the picture is, say: "My turn!" so that the child knows you are going first. Open the first door to reveal the picture and name it, e.g. "Look! **Pie**!" so that the child has an opportunity to hear you say **p** at the beginning of a short word.

3. When you have finished your go, say to the child "Your turn!" so that she knows that it is her go to open the door and name the picture behind it.

4. Put the picture of the doors over different large pictures, e.g. **pea** and **pier**, and take it in turns to open a door and name the picture behind it. Follow this procedure to name all the large pictures on the pages for this activity.

Variation

- Tell the child to close her eyes and you put a small picture of a word beginning with **p** behind each door. Then ask the child to open her eyes and open the doors. Try asking her to guess what picture is behind the door before she opens it.

Tips

*Help! The child says **bear** instead of **pear**. What can you do?*

- Don't expect the child to be able to say **p** in words immediately. Give her plenty of opportunities to hear words that begin with **p**. You could try to use the words you are working on several times in conversation, e.g. "Look! **Pear!** I like **pears.** I had a **pear** for breakfast. It was a really juicy pear. Yum!"

- Break the word into two parts and put a h in front of the vowel, e.g. **pie** = **p** + **hie**. Say the two parts leaving a pause between them: **p** (pause) – **hie**. Put two fingers on the table in a **v** shape, touch the first finger when you say **p** and touch the second finger when you say **hie**. Ask the child to copy you. Gradually they make the pause shorter and bring your fingers closer together until they are touching and there is no pause between **p** and **hie**: i.e. you are saying **pie**. Putting an h before the vowel can help the child to say **p** instead of **b** in words.

Help! The child won't try to say the words because she thinks she will make mistakes. What can you do?

- If the child gets anxious in activities and games, or is very unconfident, try using a puppet or a toy in sessions to reduce stress for her. Carry out the activities with the puppet/toy so that the child can watch and listen, but is not under any pressure to talk.

Hide the pea (Listening and speaking activity)

Aim
To provide more opportunities to say hear and say **p** at the beginning of short words: **pie**, **pear**, **paw**, **pow!**, **pier**, **pea**.

How?
By giving the child opportunities to hear, and see, you say short words that begin with **p** and to practise saying the words.

Resources

- Large pictures of short words that begin with **p**. (p. 54–56).

- Small pictures of short words that begin with **p**. (p. 57).

- Page of two doors with question marks on each one and the instruction *Close your eyes* (p. 58). You will need to copy this page and cut along three sides of the doors so that you can open them to reveal a picture.

Instructions

1. Look at the pictures with the child: "Look! A **pea**. **A pear** and a **pie!**" Read the first part of the instruction at the top of The page: "Close your eyes. I am going to hide **a pea!**" Then stick the pea on the picture of the pear or on the picture of the pie. Read the rest of the instruction to the child: "Open your eyes! Where's **the pea?**" The child has to name the picture that he thinks **the pea** is on, e.g. "**Pie!**" and then open the door to see if he is right or not. Play this game several times varying the pictures that you use.

2. Reverse the game. Say to the child: "Your turn. I'll close my eyes and you hide **the pea!**" Let the child have several turns at hiding the **pea**. To vary the pictures that you use in the game, put a small picture behind each door so that the child cannot predict what the pictures will be.

Tip

To make this a more challenging speaking game, demonstrate offering a choice of pictures when the child is listening and guessing where the pea is. For example: "Where's the pea? On pie or pear?" When you reverse the game and the child is speaking and you are listening, she has to offer you a choice, e.g. "Where's the pea? On paw or pow!?" Offering choices gives the child opportunities to say p at the beginning of more words.

Variation of the game

- If the child finds this activity hard, play it as a listening game. Tell the child to close her eyes and you place the pea on one of the pictures, e.g. **paw**. Tell the child to open her eyes and tell her where the pea is. For example: "Turn your listening ears on! Are you ready? The **pea's** on **paw**." Use a toy or puppet to play this with younger children: you tell the toy/puppet where the pea is and the child helps the toy/puppet find it.

- Show the child at least two small pictures, e.g. **pier** and **pear**. Name the pictures. Ask the child to close her eyes. Put a **pea** under one of the pictures. Ask the child to open her eyes and ask "Where's the **pea?**" The child names the picture that she thinks the pea is under, e.g. "**Pier**", and looks under the picture to see if she is right or not.

- Make more laminated pictures of a pea with velcro or Blu-tack on the back. Then show the child at least four small pictures. Name the pictures, e.g. "**Pea. Paw. Pier. Pow!**" Tell the child you are going to hide two peas! and ask her to close her eyes. Put a pea under two of the small pictures. Ask the child to open her eyes and ask "Where are the **peas**?" The child names the pictures that she thinks a pea is under, e.g. "**Paw. Pow!**" and looks under the pictures to see if she is right or not. You can increase the number of pictures and the number of peas in the game. Remember to give the child a turn at hiding a pea for you to find.

Tips

To give the child opportunities to say **p** at the beginning of more words, ask her "Where are the **peas**? Are they under **pier**, **paw**, **pie** or **pow!**?" This provides her with a model to copy when she is hiding the peas and you are finding them.

*Help! The child says **bear** instead of **pear** unless she whispers! What can you do?*

- Avoid correcting the child because that could make her feel bad about her talking. If she says **b** instead of **p** in words, e.g. **bear** instead of **pear**, say the word she wanted to say, e.g. **pear**, so that she has another chance to hear the word. Some children need lots of opportunities to hear words before they can say them.

- Say "Copy me!" to the child. Whisper, for example, "**pear**" at least five times: "**pear, pear, pear, pear, pear**". Then say "Your turn!" and the child whispers pear five times. Then say "My turn!" and whisper pear five times again, but make sure the fifth time you say **pear** you say it little bit louder than the other four. Each session, see if you can make the fifth **pear** just a fraction louder until the child is saying **pear** quietly rather than whispering.

What did I say? (Listening and speaking activity)

Aim

To say short words that begin with the speech sound **p: pie, pear, paw, pow!, pier, pea.**

How?

By giving the child opportunities to hear, and see, you say short words that begin with **p** and to practise saying the words.

Resources

- At least two sets of the small pictures of short words that begin with **p** (p. 57).

Instructions

You are the speaker and the child is the listener in these activities.

1. Choose two pictures, e.g. **pie** and **pier**. Put them on the table in front of the child and name them for her: "**Pie**. **Pier**." Tell the child to listen carefully and then you name one of the pictures in front of her, e.g. "**Pier**". Then say "What did I say?" The child listens and points to, or holds up, or puts a counter on the word she heard you say.

2. When you think the child is ready to listen and remember more words, choose three pictures, e.g. **pea**, **paw** and **pow!**. Put them on the table in front of the child and name them for her: "**Pea**. **Paw**. **Pow!**" Tell the child to listen carefully and then name two of the pictures placed in front of her: "**Pow!**. **Pea**" Then say "What did I say?" The child listens and points to, or holds up or puts a counter on the words he heard you say. Increase the number of words to make the activity more challenging when you think the child is ready. For example, choose four pictures, name them, then name three of the four and ask the child to point to the three that you said.

Variations

- To make the activity more challenging, present at least three pictures to the child. Write down the words in the order you are going to say them, not in the order they appear in front of the child. For example, the pictures in front of the child are **pow! pea**, **paw**, you might write down: **pea**, **paw**, **pow!**. Read out the words that you have written down, e.g. **pea**, **paw**, **pow!**. The child listens and arranges the pictures correspondingly, i.e. to match what you said (**pea**, **paw**, **pow!**)

- Give the same pictures to yourself and to the child. You will need at least three, e.g. **pie**, **pier**, **pow!**. Place a barrier between yourself and the child so that you cannot see each other's pictures. Arrange your pictures without the child seeing. Name the pictures in the order you have arranged them, e.g. "**Pier**. **Pow!** **Pie**." The child listens and arranges his pictures to match what you have said. Remove the barrier and see if the child's pictures are in the same order as yours! Vary the activity by, for example, giving the child four pictures but only saying three of them.

- Reverse the game so that the child is the speaker and you are the listener.

Tips

Help! The child can't remember what you said! What can you do?

- Start this activity by asking the child to remember one picture. Show her two pictures, e.g. **pea** and **pow!**, and name one of the pictures, e.g. "**Pea**". The child listens and points to the one that she heard. If she can do this easily, make the activity more challenging by presenting the child with three pictures, e.g. **pier**, **pear** and **pow!**, and naming two of them, e.g. "**Pear. Pier**". Gradually increase the number of pictures so that the child has to remember more words. If she can't remember what you said, try reducing the number of pictures you are using.

Help! The child can't write the words! What can you do?

- To take part in this activity, children have to be able to read what they have written to you, but this does not mean that they have to spell the words correctly. For example, they might write **pi** for **pie**. Ask an adult or another child to help.

- Draw pictures of the words that you are going to say to the child, instead of writing the words. The child can draw pictures of the words she is going to say in the activity. She might need some help from an adult or another child.

Help! It's really hard work to get the child to do these activities! What can you do?

- Make sure you don't do these activities for too long. If the child finds it hard to concentrate, keep the activities short and fun!

- Offer a reward to the child if she does, say, one activity. Choose a reward that you know she will enjoy, e.g. blowing bubbles, playing with Lego for five minutes. Gradually increase the number of activities she has to do in order to get the reward!

What's the word? (Listening activity)

Aim

To say short words that begin with the speech sound **p: pie, pear, paw, pow!, pier, pea**.

How?

By giving the child opportunities to hear, and see, you say short words that begin with **p** and to practise saying the words.

Resources

- At least **two sets** of the small pictures of short words that begin with **p** (p. 57).

Instructions

This activity is for children aged four and a half upwards.

1. Lay a set of the six small pictures in front of the child. Name them with the child: "**Pie. Pear. Paw. Pow!. Pier. Pea**." so that she can hear the words before you start the activity.

2. Tell the child to listen carefully and point to the picture you are naming. Break words into the first speech sound, **p**, and the vowel, e.g. "**p – ear**". Leave a short pause between **p** and the vowel to help the child carry out this task. The child has to put the **p** and the vowel together in her head to make the word, e.g. **pear**, and then point to the picture of a pear.

3. When the child is familiar with this activity, ask her to put the sounds together in her head, e.g. **p – ear**, point to the picture and say the word out loud: "**pear**". ·

Variation

• Give one set of the small pictures to yourself and one to the child. Choose at least three pictures. Do not show the child the pictures you have chosen. Place a barrier between yourself and the child so that you cannot see each other's pictures. Arrange your pictures without the child seeing them on your side of the barrier, e.g. **pow!**, **pear**, **pea**. Tell the child to listen carefully, find the pictures you say and put them on her side of the barrier. Break each word into the first sound, **p**, and the vowel, e.g. "**p – ow!, p – ear, p – ea**". The child has to put the **p** and the vowel together in her head, find the picture and put it behind her barrier. When you have finished, ask the child to say what the pictures are, e.g. "**Pow!. Pear. Pea**". Remove the barrier to see if they are the same as your pictures.

Tips

Help! The child keeps pointing to the wrong pictures! What can you do?

• This activity might be very new for the child. Help her get used to it and reduce any pressure she might be feeling, by using a toy or a puppet in the activity. Follow the instructions with the toy/puppet, so that the child can watch and listen. When the toy /puppet points to a picture, you say "Hold on a minute". Turn to the child and say, for example, "**P – ear**. Let's put them together, **P – ear, Pear**! Did he point to the **pear**? He did, didn't he? Clever puppet! He got it right!" When the child is more familiar with the activity, the toy/puppet can start to make some mistakes. For example, you say "**p**

– **aw**" and the puppet points to the picture of a pea. Check the puppet's answer with the child and see if she can help the puppet by pointing to the right picture (paw).

*Help! When the child blends **p** and **ear**, she says **bear**! What can you do?*

- This is primarily a listening activity, not a speaking activity. If the child points to the right picture, e.g. **pear**, then you know that she has blended **p** and **ear** together correctly in her head. The child said **bear** because she cannot say **p** in words yet. Say the word correctly for the child so that she has another opportunity to hear it and then ask her to repeat the word. For example: "**Pear**. [child repeats] Good work! **P – ear**. **Pear**! [child repeats] You got it!"

Roll and say (Speaking activity)

Aim

To say short words that begin with the speech sound **p**: **pie**, **pear**, **paw**, **pow!**, **pier**, **pea**.

How?

By giving the child opportunities to hear, and see, you say short words that begin with **p** and to practise saying the words.

Resources

- One set of the small pictures that have shapes on the back (photocopy the sheet of shapes (p. 26) on to the back of the pictures (p. 57)).

- A dice.

- Template for a dice with a different shape on each face (p. 27).

Instructions

1. Spread the pictures out in front of the child, face down so that you cannot see them but you can see the shapes on the back.

2. Roll the dice with shapes on it. The shapes on the dice match the shapes on the back of the pictures. Turn over the picture that has the same shape as the dice, e.g. circle, so that you can see what the picture is, e.g. **pear**.

3. Roll the dice with numbers on it. You have to say the word on your picture, e.g. **pear**, the number of times that you throw on the dice, e.g. 5: "**pear**, **pear**, **pear**, **pear**, **pear**".

Variations

- Make the game competitive: the winner is the first person to say the names of all of the six pictures in the activity, i.e. to throw all of the shapes on the dice.

- Roll the dice with shapes on it and turn over the picture that has the same shape on it, e.g. heart. Take it in turns to see how many times you can say the word in a minute. Use a one-minute salt timer.

My progress

Date	I can ...	☺/☹	I need to work on ...
	Listen carefully and hear short words that begin with **p**, e.g. **pear**, **pie**, **pier**, without any help.		
	Listen carefully and hear short words that begin with **p**, e.g. **pear**, **pie**, **pier**, with help.		
	Say **p** at the beginning of short words, e.g. **pea**, **pie**, **paw**, without any help.		
	Say **p** at the beginning of short words, e.g. **pea**, **pie**, **paw**, with some help.		

Look!

pie

pear

Look!

pow!

paw

pea

pier

Look!

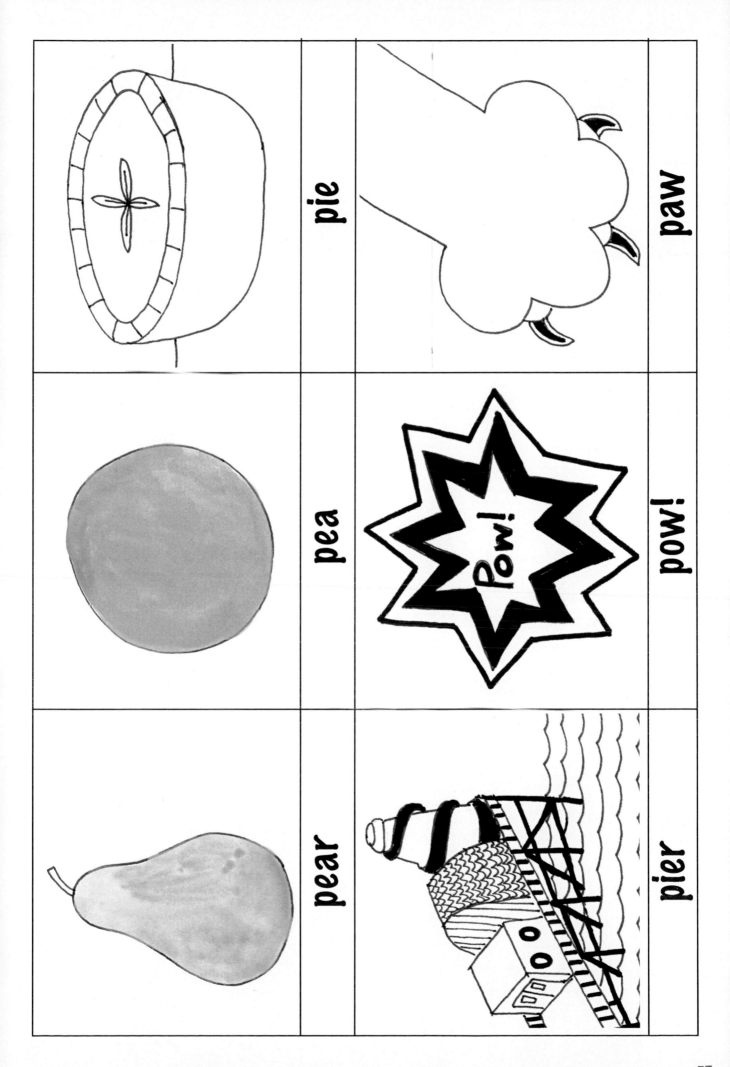

pie

paw

pea

pow!

pear

pier

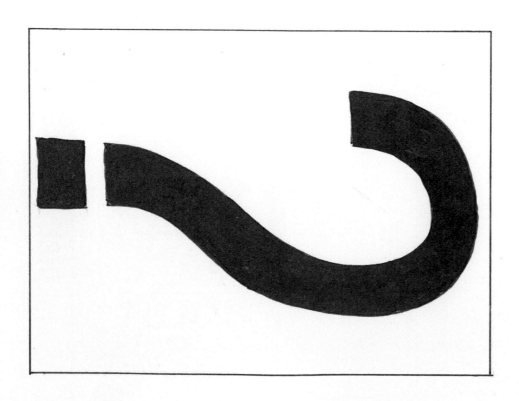

Close your eyes! I'm going to hide the pea!
Open your eyes! Where's the pea?

What's the picture? Open the door and see!

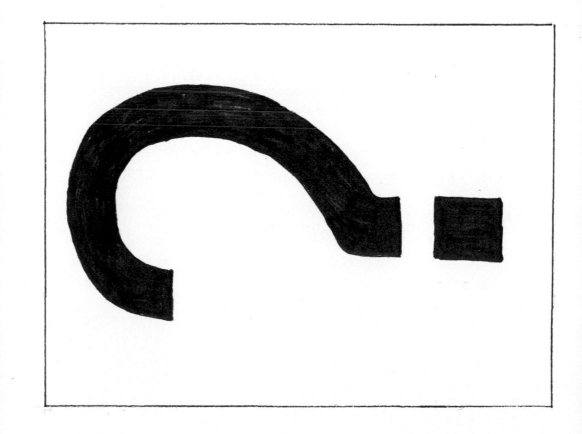

What's the next step?

I can listen carefully and hear short words that begin with **p**, e.g. **pear**, **pie**, **pier**, without any help. **Play listening games from the list of games in Section 8, e.g. Listen and colour, Catch a picture, Bowling. Start Section 4.**

I can listen carefully and hear short words that begin with **p**, e.g. **pear**, **pie**, **pier**, with help. **Carry on playing listening games from Section 3. Play listening games from the list of games in Section 8. When the child is able to listen and hear short words that begin with p without help at least 70 per cent of the time, gradually introduce listening games from Section 4.**

I can say **p** at the beginning of short words, e.g. **pea**, **pie**, **paw**, without any help. **Play speaking games from the list of games in Section 8, e.g. Pairs, Kim's game, Find the coin. Start Section 4.**

I can say **p** at the beginning of short words, e.g. **pea**, **pie**, **paw**, with some help. **Carry on playing speaking games from Section 3 and carry on doing mouth exercises from Section 1. Play games from the list of games in Section 8. When the child is able to say p at the beginning of short words that begin with p without help at least 70 per cent of the time, gradually introduce speaking games from Section 4.**

Jingles

Many children, especially young children under five, benefit from listening to words that contain the speech sound they are learning to use, in this case **p**. Listening can help raise their awareness of the speech sound in words such as **pie**, and so help them to say the speech sound.

At the end of Sections 3, 4, 5 and 6 of this book, are some jingles that contain the words you have been working on with the child, for example, in this section the short words that begin with **p**: **pea**, **pear**, **pie**, **pow!**, **paw**, **pier**.

Ideas for using the jingles

Step 1: Choose one or two jingles that contain the words you have been working on with the child.

Step 2: Read the jingle to the child and look at the pictures together.

Tip

- Use your voice to make the jingles more interesting. For example, vary your pitch – say some words in a low voice, others in a high voice; vary your volume – say some words in a loud voice, others in a quiet voice. At this stage, there is no pressure on the child to talk. She can enjoy listening to the jingles without worrying about talking.

Step 3: When the child is making progress with the speech sound you are working on, for example, she is saying **p** at the beginning of short words at least 70 per cent of the time, leave a word that contains **p** out in a line of the jingle and leave a pause to see if the child can say the missing word to complete the jingle. For example: "A **pear** on a _____ (**paw**)!" Gradually increase the number of lines in a jingle that you are doing this with. For example: "A **pear** on a _____ (**paw**)! Whose **paw** is it? A _____ (**pear**) on a dog's **paw**!" "**Pow! Paul** kicked a _____ (**pea**) Pow! _____ (**Paul**) hit a **pea**!"

Tip

- If the child cannot remember the word, sound it out for her, e.g. '**p – ear**'. See if she can put the sounds together and say the word: e.g. "**pear**".

Step 4: When the child can say the word you leave out 70 per cent of the time, try leaving out more than one word in lines to see if she can complete the jingles. For example: "Would you like _____ (**pea pie**) or _____ (**pear pie**)?"

Step 5: When the child is able to say more than one word to complete sentences (step 4), see if she can remember an entire line of a jingle! Start with short lines! For example: 'A **pear** on a **paw**! Whose **paw** is it? _____ (A **pear** on a dog's **paw**!) Try taking it in turns to say a line each of short jingles!

Step 6: Try reading jingles with older children, e.g. six to seven years old.

Jingles with short words that begin with p

Jingle one   (pictures pp.65–70)

Listen

A pear on a paw! Whose paw is it?

A pear on a dog's paw!

Two pears on a paw! Whose paw is it?

Two pears on a cat's paw!

Three pears on a paw! Whose paw is it?

Three pears on a rabbit's paw!

One pear on a dog's paw, two pears on a cat's paw, three pears on a rabbit's paw!

Say the word

A pear on a _____ (**paw**)! Whose paw is it?

A _____ (**pear**) on a dog's paw!

Two pears on a _____ (**paw**)! Whose paw is it?

Two pears on a cat's _____ (**paw**)!

Three pears on a _____ (**paw**)! Whose paw is it?

Three pears on a rabbit's _____ (**paw**)!

One pear on a dog's _____ (**paw**), two pears on a cat's _____ (**paw**), three pears on a rabbit's _____ (**paw**)!

Jingle two   (pictures pp. 71–72

Listen

Pow! Paul kicked a pea!

Pow! Paul hit a pea!

Pow! Paul threw a pea!

Pow! Paul is STRONG!

Say the word

Pow! Paul kicked a _____ (**pea**)!

Pow! Paul hit a _____ (**pea**)!

_____ (**Pow!**) Paul threw a _____ (**pea**)!

____ (**Pow!**) Paul is STRONG!

Jingle three   (pictures p. 73)

Listen

Who wants a pea?

Me!

Pea for my mum

Pea for my nan

Say the word

Who wants a _____ (**pea**)?

Me!

_____ (**Pea**) for my mum

_____ (**Pea**) for my nan

Jingle four   (pictures on pp. 74–75)

Listen

Would you like pea pie or pear pie?

Mum wants pear pie

Dad wants pea pie

Nan wants pear pie and pea pie!

Say the word

Would you like pea _____ (**pie**) or pear _____ (**pie**)?

Mum wants _____ (**pear**) pie

Dad wants _____ (**pea**) pie

Nan wants _____ (**pear**) pie and _____ (**pea**) pie!

Jingle five (picture on p. 75)

Listen

What is this? It's a poy!

A poy has one eye

A poy has two big ears

A poy has six legs with six paws

A poy has a long tail

A poy is pink!

A poy eats peas, pears and pies

This is Paul's pet poy. He is very friendly

Would you like some pie, poy?

Say the word

What is this? It's a _____ (**poy**)!

A _____ (**poy**) has one eye

A _____ (**poy**) has two big ears

A _____ (**poy**) has six legs with six paws

A _____ (**poy**) has a long tail

A _____ (**poy**) is pink!

A _____ (**poy**) eats peas, pears and pies

This is Paul's pet _____ (**poy**). He is very friendly

Would you like some _____ (**pie**), poy?

69

Look!

kick a pea

hit a pea

Look!

throw a pea

Paul is strong

look!

nan and mum

me

Look!

mum wants pear pie

dad wants pea pie

Look!

a poy has six pink paws

nan wants pea pie and pear pie

SECTION 4

SAYING P AT THE BEGINNING OF LONGER WORDS

Section 4: **Saying p at the beginning of longer words**

What's the picture? (Speaking activity)

Aim
To say longer words that begin with the speech sound **p**: **pipe**, **pot**, **pig**, **pan**, **pin**, **park**, **pill**, **purse**, **peach**, **Paul**.

How?
By giving the child opportunities to hear, and see, you say longer words that begin with **p** and to practise saying the words.

Resources
- Large pictures of longer words that begin with the speech sound **p**: (pp. 88–92).

- Small pictures of longer words that begin with the speech sound **p**: (pp. 93–94)

- Page of two doors with question marks on each one and the instruction *What's the picture?* (p. 59). You will need to photocopy this page and cut along three sides of the doors so that you can open them to reveal a picture.

Instructions
1. Put the page with the doors on top of large pictures of longer words that begin with **p**, e.g. **pill** and **park**.

2. Read the instruction at the top of the page to the child: *What's the picture? Open the door and see.* Before you open the door to see what the picture is, say "My turn!" so that the child knows you are going first. Open the first door to reveal the picture and name it, e.g. "Look! **Park**!" so that the child has an opportunity to hear you say **p** at the beginning of a longer word.

3. When you have finished your go, say to the child "Your turn!" so that he knows that it is his go to open the door and name the picture behind it.

4. Put the picture of the doors over different large pictures, e.g. **pan**! and **pin**, and take it in turns to open a door and name the picture behind it. Follow this procedure to name all the pictures on the pages for this activity.

Variation
- Tell the child to close his eyes and you put a small picture of a longer word beginning with **p** behind each door. Then ask the child to open his eyes and open the doors. Try asking him to guess what picture is behind the door before he opens it.

Roll and say (Speaking activity)

Aim

To say longer words that begin with the speech sound **p: pipe**, **pot**, **pig**, **pan**, **pin**, **park**, **pill**, **purse**, **peach**, **Paul**.

How?

By giving the child opportunities to hear, and see, you say longer words that begin with **p** and to practise saying the words.

Resources

- One set of the small pictures that have shapes on the back (photocopy the sheet of shapes (p. 26) on to the back of the picture) (p. 93, 94).

- A dice.

- Template for a dice with a different shape on each face (p. 27).

Instructions

1. Spread the pictures out in front of the child, six at a time, face down so that you cannot see them but you can see the shapes on the back.

2. Roll the dice with shapes on it. The shapes on the dice match the shapes on the back of the pictures. Turn over the picture that has the same shape as the dice, e.g. circle, so that you can see what the picture is, e.g. **pig**.

3. Roll the dice with numbers on it. You have to say the word on your picture, e.g. **pig**, the number of times that you throw on the dice, e.g. 5: "**pig, pig, pig, pig, pig**" Make sure you have the first turn so that you can demonstrate the activity to the child.

Variations

- Make the game competitive: the winner is the first person to say the names of all of the six pictures in the activity, i.e. to throw all of the shapes on the dice.

- Roll the dice with shapes on it and turn over the picture that has the same shape on it, e.g. heart. Take it in turns to see how many times you can say the word in a minute. Use a one-minute salt timer.

Remember and say (Listening and speaking activity)

Aim

To say longer words that begin with the speech sound **p**: **pipe**, **pot**, **pig**, **pan**, **pin**, **park**, **pill**, **purse**, **peach**, **Paul**.

How?

By giving the child opportunities to hear, and see, you say words that begin with **p** and to practise saying the words.

Resources

- At least one set of the small pictures of words that begin with **p**: (pp. 93–94)

Instructions

1. Look at the pictures of the longer words that begin with **p** and name them with the child.

2. Present at least two of the small pictures to the child and name them, e.g. "**Pot. Pill**". Tell the child to "take a photo"of the pictures in his mind, i.e. use a mental camera, to help him remember them. Give him at least 30 seconds to look at the pictures. Then turn the pictures over and ask the child if he can remember what they are. The child then names the pictures. Turn them over to see if he is right. Make this activity more challenging by increasing the number of pictures that the child has to remember.

Variations

- Give the same pictures to yourself and to the child. You will need at least four, e.g. **Paul**, **purse**, **peach**, **pan**. Place a barrier between yourself and the child so that you cannot see each other's pictures. Arrange at least two of your pictures behind the barrier so that the child cannot see what they are. Name the pictures, e.g. "**Purse. Pan**". Pause for a few seconds and then say: "Ready, Steady, Go!" The child listens, then looks at his pictures, finds the ones he heard you name and lays them out on his side of the barrier. When you remove the barrier you will see if the child's pictures are the same as yours! Reverse the game so that the child names pictures for you to remember and arrange behind the barrier.

- Play Kim's game with the pictures (see instructions in Section 8 p. 193).

- Play Pairs (see instructions in Section 8 p. 193).

Listen and guess (Listening and speaking activity)

Aim

To say longer words that begin with the speech sound **p**: **pipe**, **pot**, **pig**, **pan**, **pin**, **park**, **pill**, **purse**, **peach**, **Paul**.

How?

By giving the child opportunities to hear, and see, you say words that begin with **p** and to practise saying the words.

Resources

• One set of the small pictures of longer words that begin with **p** (pp. 93–94).

Instructions

1. Choose a picture, e.g. **purse**. Do not show it to the child. Place it face down in front of him.

2. Tell the child at least three things about the picture, e.g. "You put money in it. You keep it in your handbag. It is often made of leather."

3. The child guesses what the picture is and turns it over to see if he is right. **Reverse** the game so that the child chooses a picture and describes it and you guess what it is.

Variations

• To make this activity less challenging for the child, put at least three pictures in front of him, e.g. **purse**, **park**, **pipe**. Choose one of the pictures to describe, e.g. **park**, but do not tell the child which picture you have chosen. Tell him three things about the picture, e.g. "Children go there to play. You can go on swings and slides there. Some of these have cafes." The child listens and points to the picture that he thinks you are describing, e.g. **park**.

• To make this activity more challenging, choose at least three pictures. Do not show them to the child. Place them face down in front of him. Tell the child at least three things about the first picture. The child guesses what it is and turns it over to see if he is right or not. Then tell him three things about the second picture. The child guesses and checks if he is right or not. Follow the same procedure for the third picture. Reverse the game, so that the child chooses at least three pictures and describes them to you.

- Place a barrier between you and the child. Make sure that you and the child have a set of the small pictures. Choose at least three pictures from your set, e.g. **park**, **peach**, **pig**. Describe the pictures to the child leaving a pause between each description so that he can find the picture he thinks you are talking about in his set. When the child has found the picture he thinks you are describing, he puts it face up behind the barrier so that you cannot see it. When you have described all three pictures and the child has put three corresponding pictures behind the barrier, ask him to say what his pictures are, e.g. "**park**. **peach**. **pig**". Then remove the barrier to see if he has the same pictures as you. Reverse the game, so that the child chooses and describes his pictures and you listen and try to find the corresponding picture in your set.

What did I say? (Listening and speaking activity)

Aim

To say longer words that begin with the speech sound **p**: **pipe**, **pot**, **pig**, **pan**, **pin**, **park**, **pill**, **purse**, **peach**, **Paul**.

How?

By giving the child opportunities to hear, and see, you say longer words that begin with **p** and to practise saying the words.

Resources

- At least two sets of the small pictures of longer words that begin with **p** (pp. 93–94)

Instructions

You are the speaker and the child is the listener in these activities.

1. Choose two pictures, e.g. **pan** and **pig**. Put them on the table in front of the child and name them for him: "**Pan. Pig**" Tell the child to listen carefully and then you name one of the pictures placed in front of him, e.g. "**Pig**". Then say "What did I say?" The child listens and points to, or holds up, or puts a counter on the picture of the word he heard you say.

2. When you think the child is ready to listen and remember more words, choose three pictures, e.g. **pill**, **pipe** and **pot**. Put them on the table in front of the child and name them for him: "**Pill. Pipe. Pot**". Tell the child to listen carefully and then you name two of the pictures in front of him, e.g. "**Pot. Pill**". Then say "What did I say?" The child listens and points to, or holds up, or puts a counter on the words he heard you say. Increase the number of words to make the activity more challenging when you think

the child is ready. For example, choose four pictures, name them, then name three of the four and ask the child to point to the three that you said.

Variations

• To make the activity more challenging, present at least three pictures to the child. Write down the words in the order you are going to say them, not in the order they appear in front of the child. For example, if the pictures in front of the child are **pill**, **pipe**, **pot**, you might write down **pot**, **pill**, **pipe**. Read out the words that you have written down: **pot**, **pill**, **pipe**. The child listens and arranges the pictures correspondingly, i.e. to match what you said (**pot**, **pill**, **pipe**).

• Give the same pictures to yourself and to the child. You will need at least three, e.g. **Paul**, **purse**, **park**. Place a barrier between yourself and the child so that you cannot see each other's pictures. Arrange your pictures without the child seeing. Name the pictures in the order you have arranged them, e.g. '**Park. Paul. Purse**'. The child listens and arranges his pictures to match what you have said. Remove the barrier and see if the child's pictures are in the same order as yours!

• Reverse the game so that the child is the speaker and you are the listener.

Tips

Help! The child can't remember what you said! What can you do?

• Start this activity by asking the child to remember one picture. Show him two pictures, e.g. **pot** and **purse**, and name one of the pictures, e.g. "**Pot**". The child listens and points to the one that he heard. If he can do this easily, make the activity more challenging by presenting the child with three pictures, e.g. **pin**, **pan**, **pig**, and naming two of them, e.g. "**Pan. Pig**". Gradually increase the number of pictures so that the child has to remember more words. If he cannot remember what you said, try reducing the number of pictures you are using.

Help! The child can't write the words! What can you do?

• To take part in this activity, children have to be able to read what they have written to you, but this does not mean that they have to spell the words correctly. For example: they might write '**pers**' for '**purse**'. Ask an adult or another child to help.

• Draw pictures of the words that you are going to say to the child, instead of writing the words. The child can draw pictures of the words he is going to say in the activity. He might need some help from an adult or another child.

Help! It's really hard work to get the child to do these activities! What can you do?

- Make sure you don't do these activities for too long. If the child finds it hard to concentrate, keep them short and fun!

- Offer a reward to the child if he does, say, one activity. Choose a reward that you know he will enjoy, e.g. blowing bubbles, playing with Lego for five minutes. Gradually increase the number of activities he has to do in order to get the reward!

What's the word? (Listening activity)

Aim
To say longer words that begin with the speech sound **p**: **pipe, pot, pig, pan, pin, park, pill, purse, peach, Paul.**

How?
By giving the child opportunities to hear, and see, you say longer words that begin with **p** and to practise saying the words.

Resources
- At least two sets of the small pictures of longer words that begin with **p** (pp. 93–94)

Instructions

This activity is for children aged four and a half upwards.

1. Lay a set of the small pictures in front of the child. Name them with the child so that he can hear the words before you start the activity.

2. Tell the child to listen carefully and point to the picture you are naming. Break words into the first speech sound, **p**, and the rest of the word, e.g. "**p – ot**". Leave a short pause between the speech sounds to help the child carry out this task. The child has to put the speech sounds together in his head to make the word, e.g. **pot**, and then point to the picture of a pot.

3. When the child is familiar with this activity, ask him to put the sounds together in his head, e.g. **p – ot**, point to the picture and say the word out loud, e.g. "**pot**".

Variations
- Give one set of the ten small pictures to yourself and one to the child. Choose at least three. Do not show the child the pictures you have chosen. Place a barrier between yourself and the child so that you cannot see each other's pictures. Arrange your pictures without the child seeing them on your side of the barrier, e.g. **pan, park, pill.** Tell the child to listen carefully, find the pictures you say and put them on his side of

the barrier. Break each word into the first sound, **p**, and the rest of the word, e.g. "**p –
an**, **p – ark**, **p – ill**". The child has to put the speech sounds together in his head, find
the picture and put it behind his barrier. When you have finished, ask the child to say
what the pictures are, e.g. "**Pan. Park. Pill**". Remove the barrier to see if they are the
same as your pictures.

• Challenge older children by breaking words into three parts, e.g. **p – o – t, p – a – n**.

Tips

Help! The child keeps pointing to the wrong pictures! What can you do?

• This activity might be very new for the child. Help him get used to it and reduce any
pressure he might be feeling, by using a toy or a puppet. Follow the instructions with
the toy/puppet, so that the child can watch and listen. When the toy/puppet points to
a picture, you say, "Hold on a minute". Turn to the child and say, for example: "**P – ark**.
Let's put them together. **P – ark. Park!** Did he point to the **park**? He did, didn't he?
Clever puppet! He got it right!" When the child is more familiar with the activity, the
puppet/toy can start to make some mistakes. For example, you say
"**p – an**" and the puppet points to the picture of a pot. Check the puppet's answer
with the child and see if he can help the puppet by pointing to the right picture (pan).

*Help! When the child tries to say longer words that begin with **p**, e.g. **park**, he says **b**! He
says **bark** instead of **park**! What can you do?*

• This is primarily a listening activity, not a speaking activity. If the child points to the
right picture, e.g. **park**, then you know that he has blended **p** and **ark** together
correctly in his head. The child said **bark** because he cannot say **p** in words yet. Say
the word correctly for the child so that he has another opportunity to hear it. For
example: "**Park.** [child repeats] Good work! **P – ark. Park!** [child repeats] You got it!"

*How can you help the child to say **p** in words?*

• You will need two coins or Lego bricks and small pictures of the words that you are
working on with the child, e.g. **park, pill, pot, pan**. Choose one of the pictures,
e.g. **park**. Put the two coins or Lego bricks in front of the child, leaving a gap between
the two objects. Touch the first coin or brick and say the first sound of the word: **p**.
Then touch the second coin or brick and say the rest of the word: **ark (park)**. Take it in
turns to touch the coins or bricks and say **p** and **ark** as you touch each one. Gradually
move the two objects closer together so that the pause you leave between saying **p**
and saying **ark** is smaller and smaller, until the coins or bricks are touching and there
is no gap between **p** and **ark**, i.e. you are saying **park**.

• Instead of asking the child to say **p – ark**, try asking him to say **par**, leave a pause and then say **k** (**par – k**). Saying a speech sound and doing a movement, e.g. touching a brick, touching one of your fingers, jumping on a mat, helps some children to say words. Use coins or bricks as described in the first tip. Or try putting two mats or pieces of paper or paper footprints on the floor for the child to step or jump on when he says **par** and **k**. Or try putting paper hands on a wall for the child to touch when he says **par** and **k**. Gradually bring the two mats or pieces of paper together until they are touching and there is no gap between **par** and **k**, i.e. you are saying **park**.

My progress

Date	I can ...	☺/☹	I need to work on ...
	Listen carefully and hear words that begin with **p**, e.g. **pan**, **pot**, **pig**, without any help.		
	listen carefully and hear words that begin with **p**, e.g. **pan**, **pot**, **pig**, with help.		
	say **p** at the beginning of words, e.g. **pill**, **pin**, **park**, without any help.		
	say **p** at the beginning of words, e.g. **pill**, **pin**, **park**, with some help.		

Look!

pan

pin

look!

pig

pot

pipe

Paul

Look!

Look!

peach

purse

Look!

pill

park

pot

pin

park

pan

pill

pig

peach

Paul

purse

pipe

What's the next step?

- I can listen carefully and hear words that begin with **p**, e.g. **pan**, **pot**, **pig**, without any help. **Start doing listening activities in Section 5. Play listening games from the list of games in Section 8, e.g. Goal! Listen and colour.**

- I can listen carefully and hear words that begin with **p**, **e.g. pan**, **pot**, **pig**, with help. **Carry on doing listening activities in Section 4. Use games from Section 2 and play listening games from Section 8, e.g. Bowling, Catch a picture. Start introducing listening activities from Section 5 when the child can hear words that begin with p in activities at least 70 per cent of the time.**

- I can say **p** at the beginning of words, e.g. **pill**, **pin**, **park**, without any help. **Start working on Section 5. Play speaking games from the list of games in Section 8, e.g. Guess what? What is it?**

- I can say **p** at the beginning of words, e.g. **pill**, **pin**, **park**, with some help. **Carry on playing speaking games from Section 4 and carry on doing mouth exercises from Section 1. Play games from the list of games in Section 8. When the child is able to say p at the beginning of longer words that begin with p without help at least 70 per cent of the time, gradually introduce speaking games from Section 5.**

Jingles with words that begin with p

See advice at the end of Section 3 on how to use the jingles in sessions (pp. 60–61)

Jingle one   (pictures pp. 99–100)

Listen

Pig! Don't push Paul in the pool!

Pig! Don't push Pam in the pool!

Paul and Pam don't push pig in the pool!

He can't swim!

Say the word

Pig! Don't push Paul in the _____ (**pool**)!

Pig! Don't _____ (**push**) Pam in the pool!

Paul and Pam don't push _____ (**pig**) in the pool!

He can't swim!

Jingle two (pictures pp. 100–102)

Listen

Pat a pig!

Poke a pig!

Push a pig!

Pack a pig!

Poor pig!

Say the word

_____ (**Pat**) a pig!

_____ (**Poke**) a pig!

_____ (**Push**) a pig!

_____ (**Pack**) a pig!

Poor _____ (**pig**)!

Jingle three (picture p. 103)

Listen

Paul likes peach

Paul likes peach in the park

Paul likes peach in the pool in the park

Paul likes peach in the pub while dad has a pint of beer!

Say the word

Paul likes _____ (**peach**)

Paul likes peach in the _____ (**park**)

Paul likes peach in the _____ (**pool**) in the park

Paul likes _____ (**peach**) in the pub while his dad has a pint of beer!

Jingle four (pictures pp. 104–106)

Listen

Put it in Pam's purse

Put it in Pat's pot

Put it in Paul's pan

Poke it!

Push it!

Pop it!

Pam, Pat, Paul! Put it in the bin!

Say the word

Put it in Pam's _____ (**purse**)

Put it in Pat's _____ (**pot**)

Put it in Paul's _____ (**pan**)

_____ (**Poke**) it!

_____ (**Push**) it!

_____ (**Pop**) it!

Pam, Pat, _____ (**Paul**)! Put it in the bin!

Jingle five (pictures p. 107)

Listen

There is a pip in the peach, Paul

There is a pip in the peach in the park, Paul

There is a pip in the peach in the pool in the park, Paul

There is a pip in the peach in a purse in the pool in the park, Paul

There is a pip in the peach in Pam's purse in the pool in the park, Paul

Say the word

There is a pip in the _____ (**peach**), Paul

There is a pip in the peach in the _____ (**park**), Paul

There is a pip in the peach in the _____ (**pool**) in the park, Paul

There is a pip in the peach in a _____ (**purse**) in the pool in the park, Paul

There is a pip in the peach in _____ (**Pam's**) purse in the pool in the park, Paul

Look!

Pig! Don't push Pam!

Pig! Don't push Paul!

Look!

Don't push a pig!

Pat a pig!

Look!

Push a pig!

Poke a pig!

Look!

Pack a pig!

Poor pig!

Paul likes peach

Look!

Pam's purse

Pat's pot

Look!

Poke it!

Paul's pan

Look!

Push it!

Pop it!

Look!

a pip in a peach

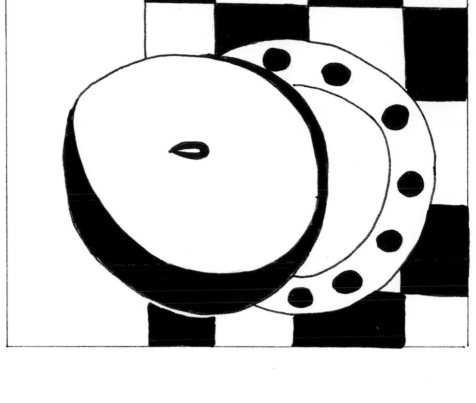

a pip in a peach in Pam's purse

SECTION 5

SAYING P AT THE END OF WORDS

Section 5: Saying p at the end of words

What's the picture? (Speaking activity)

Aim

To say longer words that end with the speech sound **p**: **mop**, **map**, **tap**, **cup**, **ship**, **sheep**, **cap**, **lip**, **hop**, **jump**, **chip**, **soap**, **soup**, **zip**.

How?

By giving the child opportunities to hear, and see, you say longer words that end with **p** and to practise saying the words.

Resources

- Large pictures of longer words that end with the speech sound **p** (pp. 120–126)

- Small pictures of longer words that begin with the speech sound **p** (pp. 127–129)

- Page of two doors with question marks on each one and the instruction *What's the picture?* (p. 59). You will need to photocopy this page and cut along three sides of the doors so that you can open them to reveal a picture.

Instructions

1. Put the page with the doors on top of large pictures of words that end with p, e.g. **cup** and **cap**.

2. Read the instruction at the top of the page to the child: *What's the picture? Open the door and see.* Before you open the door to see what the picture is, say "My turn!" so the child knows you are going first. Open the first door to reveal the picture and name it, e.g. "Look! **Cup!**" so that the child has an opportunity to hear you say **p** at the end of the word.

3. When you have finished your go, say to the child "Your turn!" so that she knows that it is her go to open the door and name the picture behind it.

4. Put the picture of the doors over different large pictures, e.g. **hop** and **jump**, and take it in turns to open a door and name the picture behind it. Follow this procedure to name all the pictures on the pages for this activity.

Variation

- Tell the child to close her eyes and you put a small picture of a word that ends with **p** behind each door. Then ask the child to open her eyes and open the doors. Try asking her to guess what picture is behind the door before she opens it.

Roll and say (Speaking activity)

Aim

To say longer words that end with the speech sound **p: mop**, **map**, **tap**, **cup**, **ship**, **sheep**, **cap**, **lip**, **hop**, **jump**, **chip**, **soap**, **soup**, **zip**.

How?

By giving the child opportunities to hear, and see, you say words that end with **p** and to practise saying the words.

Resources

- One set of the small pictures that have shapes on the back (photocopy the sheet of shapes (p. 26) on to the back of the pictures (pp. 127–129)).

- A dice.

- Template for a dice with a different shape on each face (p. 27).

Instructions

1. Spread the pictures out in front of the child, six at a time, face down so that you cannot see them but you can see the shapes on the back.
2. Roll the dice with shapes on it. The shapes on the dice match the shapes on the back of the pictures. Turn over the picture that has the same shape as the dice, e.g. circle, so that you can see what the picture is, e.g. **mop**.
3. Roll the dice with numbers on it. You have to say the word on your picture, e.g. **mop**, the number of times that you throw on the dice, e.g. 5: "**mop**, **mop**, **mop**, **mop**, **mop**." Make sure you have the first turn so that you can demonstrate the activity to the child.

Variations

- Make the game competitive: the winner is the first person to say the names of all of the six pictures in the activity, i.e. to throw all of the shapes on the dice.

- Roll the dice with shapes on it and turn over the picture that has the same shape on it, e.g. heart. Take it in turns to see how many times you can say the word in a minute. Use a one-minute salt timer.

Remember and say (Listening and speaking activity)

Aim

To say longer words that end with the speech sound **p**: **mop**, **map**, **tap**, **cup**, **ship**, **sheep**, **cap**, **lip**, **hop**, **jump**, **chip**, **soap**, **soup**, **zip**.

How?

By giving the child opportunities to hear, and see, you say words that end with **p** and to practise saying the words.

Resources

- At least one set of the small pictures of words that end with **p** (pp. 127–129)

Instructions

1. Look at the pictures of the words that end with **p** and name them with the child.

Tips

- Use at least three pictures with younger children. Be flexible with the number of pictures you present at the beginning of the activity depending on the level of the child.
- Avoid using pictures of words that contain speech sounds the child cannot yet say in speaking activities. For example, most children usually start using the speech sounds **s** and **f** in their talking at between two and a half and three years of age, the speech sound **l** between the age of three and three and a half, and **sh** between three and a half and four years of age (Grunwell, 1985).

2. Present at least two of the pictures to the child and name them, e.g. "**Mop. Tap**". Tell the child to "take a photo" of the pictures in her mind, i.e. use a mental camera, to help her remember them. Give her at least 30 seconds to look at the pictures. Then turn the pictures over and ask the child if she can remember what they are. The child then names the pictures. Turn them over to see if she is right. Make this activity more challenging by increasing the number of pictures that the child has to remember.

Variations

- Give the same pictures to yourself and to the child. You will need at least four, e.g. **mop**, **tap**, **cup**, **ship**. Place a barrier between yourself and the child so that you cannot see each other's pictures. Arrange at least two of your pictures behind the barrier so that the child cannot see what they are. Name the pictures, e.g. "**Tap**. **Ship**". Pause for a few seconds and then say: "Ready, Steady, Go!" The child listens, then looks at her pictures, finds the ones she heard you name and lays them out on her side of the barrier. When you remove the barrier you will see if the child's pictures are the same as yours! Reverse the game so that the child names pictures for you to remember and arrange behind the barrier.

• Play Kim's game with the small pictures (see instructions in Section 8 p.193).

• Play Pairs (see instructions in Section 8 p. 193).

Listen and guess (Listening and speaking activity)

Aim

To say longer words that end with the speech sound **p: mop**, **map**, **tap**, **cup**, **ship**, **sheep**, **cap**, **lip**, **hop**, **jump**, **chip**, **soap**, **soup**, **zip**.

How?

By giving the child opportunities to hear, and see, you say words that end with **p** and to practise saying the words.

Resources

• One set of the small pictures of words that end with **p** (pp. 127–129).

Instructions

1. Choose a picture, e.g. **soap**. Do not show it to the child. Place it face down in front of her.
2. Tell the child at least three things about the picture, e.g. "You find it in the bathroom. You wash your hands with it. It smells nice."
3. The child guesses what the picture is and turns it over to see if she is right. Reverse the game so that the child chooses a picture and describes it and you guess what it is.

Variations

• To make this activity less challenging for the child, put at least three pictures in front of her, e.g. **sheep**, **cap**, **tap**. Choose one of the pictures to describe, e.g. **ship**. Do not tell the child which one you have chosen. Tell her three things about the picture, e.g. "It is an animal. It eats grass. We make jumpers out of its coat." The child listens and points to the picture that she thinks you are describing, e.g. **sheep**.

- To make this activity more challenging, choose at least three pictures. Do not show them to the child. Place them face down in front of her. Tell the child at least three things about the first picture. The child guesses what it is and turns it over to see if she is right or not. Then tell her three things about the second picture. The child guesses and checks if she is right or not. Follow the same procedure for the third picture. Reverse the game, so that the child chooses at least three pictures and describes them to you.

- Place a barrier between you and the child. Make sure that you and the child each have a set of the small pictures. Choose at least three pictures from your set, e.g. **chip**, **cup**, **mop**. Describe the pictures to the child, leaving a pause between each description so that she can find the picture she thinks you are talking about in her set. When the child has found the picture she thinks you are describing, she puts it face up behind the barrier so that you cannot see it. When you have described all three pictures and the child has put three corresponding pictures behind the barrier, ask her to say what her pictures are, e.g. "**chip**, **cup**, **mop**". Then remove the barrier to see if she has the same pictures as you. Reverse the game, so that the child chooses and describes her pictures and you listen and try to find the corresponding picture in your set.

What did I say? (Listening and speaking activity)

Aim
To say longer words that end with the speech sound **p**: **mop**, **map**, **tap**, **cup**, **ship**, **sheep**, **cap**, **lip**, **hop**, **jump**, **chip**, **soap**, **soup**, **zip**.

How?
By giving the child opportunities to hear, and see, you say longer words that end with **p** and to practise saying the words.

Resources
- At least two sets of the small picture of words that end with **p** (pp. 127–129).

Instructions
You are the speaker and the child is the listener in these activities.
1. Choose two pictures, e.g. **chip** and **map**. Put them on the table in front of the child and name them for her: "**Chip**. **Map**" Tell the child to listen carefully and then you name one of the pictures in front of her, e.g. "**Map**". Then say "What did I say?" The child listens and points to, or holds up, or puts a counter on the word she heard you say.

2. When you think the child is ready to listen and remember more words, choose three pictures, e.g. **soap**, **cup** and **zip**. Put them on the table in front of the child and name them for her: "**Soap**. **Cup**. **Zip**". Tell the child to listen carefully and then you name two of the pictures in front of her, e.g. "**Cup**. **Soap**". Then say "What did I say?" The child listens and points to, or holds up, or puts a counter on the words she heard you say. Increase the number of words to make the activity more challenging when you think the child is ready. For example, choose four pictures, name them, then name three of the four and ask the child to point to the three that you said.

See variations and tips for this activity in Section 4.

Tips

Help! The child can't remember what you said! What can you do?

- Start this activity by asking the child to remember one picture. Show her two pictures, e.g. **map** and **sheep** and name one of the pictures, e.g. "**Sheep**". The child listens and points to the one that he heard. If she can do this easily, make the activity more challenging by presenting the child with three pictures, e.g. **map**, **sheep**, **cap**, and naming two of them, e.g. "**Sheep**, **Cap**". Gradually increase the number of pictures so that the she has to remember more words. If she cannot remember what you said, try reducing the number of pictures you are using.

Help! The child can't write the words! What can you do?

- To take part in this activity, children have to be able to read what they have written to you, but this does not mean that they have to spell the words correctly. For example: they might write **sop** for **soap**. Ask an adult or another child to help.

- Draw pictures of the words that you are going to say to the child, instead of writing the words. The child can draw pictures of the words she is going to say in the activity. She might need some help from an adult or another child.

Help! It's really hard work to get the child to do these activities! What can you do?

- Make sure you don't do these activities for too long. If the child finds it hard to concentrate, keep them short and fun!

- Offer a reward to the child if she does, say, one activity. Choose a reward that you know she will enjoy, e.g. blowing bubbles, playing with Lego for five minutes. Gradually increase the number of activities she has to do in order to get the reward!

What's the word? (Listening activity)

Aim

To say longer words that end with the speech sound **p**: **mop**, **map**, **tap**, **cup**, **ship**, **sheep**, **cap**, **lip**, **hop**, **jump**, **chip**, **soap**, **soup**, **zip**.

How?

By giving the child opportunities to hear, and see, you say words that end with **p** and to practise saying the words.

Resources

- At least two sets of the small picture of words that end with **p** (pp. 127–129)

Instructions

This activity is for children aged four and a half upwards.

1. Lay a set of the small pictures in front of the child. Name them with the child so that he can hear the words before you start the activity.

Tips

- Use at least three small pictures with younger children. Be flexible with the number of pictures you present at the beginning of the activity depending on the level of the child.

- Some children may have other speech sound difficulties, for example they may say **t** instead of **k** in words: **tup** instead of **cup**. However, you are working on saying **p** in words, so this is the only speech sound you need to focus on in these activities.

2. Tell the child to listen carefully and point to the picture you are naming. Break words into two parts, e.g. **ma – p**. Leave a short pause between the speech sounds to help the child carry out this task. The child has to put the speech sounds together in her head to make the word, e.g. **map**, and then point to the picture of a map.

3. When the child is familiar with this activity, ask her to put the sounds together in their head, e.g. **ma – p**, point to the picture and say the word out loud: "**map**"

See Section 4 for ideas for variations of this activity, which you can play with the words in Section 5.

Tips

*How can you help the child to say **p** at the end of words?*

- You will need two coins or Lego bricks and small pictures of the words that you are working on with the child, e.g. **hop**, **map**, **cup**. Choose one of the pictures, e.g. **map**. Put the two coins or Lego bricks in front of the child, leaving a gap between the two objects. Touch the first coin or brick and say the first part of the word, e.g. **ma**. Then touch the second coin or brick and say the final speech sound, e.g. **p** (**ma – p**). Take it in turns to touch the coins or bricks and say **ma** and **p** as you touch each one. Gradually move the two objects closer together so that the pause you leave between saying **ma** and saying **p** is smaller and smaller, until the coins or bricks are touching and there is no gap between **ma** and **p**, i.e. you are saying **map**.

My progress

Date	I can ...	☺/☹	I need to work on ...
	Listen carefully and hear words that end with **p**, e.g. **cap**, **mop**, **sheep**, without any help.		
	Listen carefully and hear words that end with **p**, e.g. **cap**, **mop**, **sheep**, with help.		
	Say **p** at the end of words, e.g. **tap**, **chip**, **cup**, without any help.		
	Say **p** at the end of words, e.g. **tap**, **chip**, **cup**, with some help.		

What's the next step?

- I can listen carefully and hear words that end with **p**, e.g. **cap**, **mop**, **sheep**, without any help. **Continue to play listening games from the list of games in Section 8. Start working on Section 6: I can say p at the beginning of longer words, e.g. pizza, pepper, poodle**.

- I can listen carefully and hear words that end with **p**, e.g. **cap**, **mop**, **sheep**, with help. **Keep playing listening games from Section 5. Play listening games from earlier sections to revise listening to p in words and listening games from the list of games in Section 8, e.g. Listen and do. When the child can hear words that end with p at least 70 per cent of the time in listening games, start working on listening games in Section 6.**

- I can say p at the end of words, e.g. **tap**, **chip**, **cup**, without any help. **Start working on speaking activities in Section 6. Play speaking games from the list of games in Section 8, e.g. Pairs, Kim's game.**

- I can say p at the end of words, e.g. **tap**, **chip**, **cup**, with some help. **Continue doing speaking activities from Section 5. Play speaking games from the list of games in Section 8. When the child can say words that end with p at least 70 per cent of the time in speaking games, start working on listening games in Section 6.**

hop

jump

Look!

Look!

map

sheep

mop

soap

Look!

122

Look!

soup

chip

tap

ship

Look!

124

Look!

zip

lip

Look!

cup

cap

cup

jump

map

hop

sheep

cap

127

soup

chip

zip

soap

lip

mop

ship

tap

Jingles with words that end with p

See advice at the end of Section 3 on how to use the jingles in sessions (pp. 60–61).

Jingle one

Listen

Pim pom pump
Do a big jump
Pim pom pump
Do a little jump
Pip pap pop
Do a big hop
Pip pap pop
Do a little hop

Say the word

Pim pom _____ (**pump**)
Do a big _____ (**jump**)
Pim pom _____ (**pump**)
Do a little _____ (**jump**)
Pip pap _____ (**pop**)
Do a big _____ (**hop**)
Pip pap _____ (**pop**)
Do a little _____ (**hop**)

Jingle two   (pictures p. 133)

Listen

Have you ever seen a sheep eat a chip?
Have you ever seen a sheep eat soup?
Have you ever seen a sheep wear a cap?
Have you ever seen a sheep looking at a map?
No. Have you?
No.

Say the word

Have you ever seen a sheep eat a _____ (**chip**)?
Have you ever seen a sheep eat _____ (**soup**)?

Have you ever seen a sheep wear a _____ (**cap**)?

Have you ever seen a sheep looking at a _____ (**map**)?

No. Have you?

No.

Jingle three (picture p. 134)

Listen

Hey! That sheep's wearing my cap!

Give it back, sheep!

Hey! That sheep's eating my soup and my chip!

Give it back, sheep!

Hey! That sheep's looking at my map!!

Give it back, sheep!

What a naughty sheep!

Say the word

Hey! That sheep's wearing my _____ (**cap**)!

Give it back, _____ (**sheep**)!

Hey! That sheep's eating my _____ (**soup**) and my _____ (**chip**)!

Give it back, _____ (**sheep**)!

Hey! That sheep's looking at my _____ (**map**)!

Give it back, _____ (**sheep**)!

What a naughty _____ (**sheep**)!

Jingle four (picture p. 135)

Listen

Bee bop beep

I'm counting sheep

One, two, three, four

Jump up and mop the floor

Five, six, seven, eight

Put a chip on my plate

I'm counting sheep

Say the word

Bee bop _____ (**beep**)

I'm counting _____ (**sheep**)

One, two, three, four

Jump up and _____ (**mop**) the floor

Five, six, seven, eight

Put a _____ (**chip**) on my plate

I'm counting sheep

SECTION 6

SAYING P
IN LONGER WORDS

Section 6: Saying p in longer words

Look and guess (Speaking activity)

Aim

To say longer words that begin with the speech sound **p**, **pizza**, **pepper**, **poodle**, **puppy**, **poppy**, **paper**, **pillow**, **pebble**, **puddle**, **purple**, **popper**, **people**, **pasta**, **panda**, **pink**, **paint**, **pencil**, **parcel**, **pocket**, **pancake**, **peanut**, **pelican**, **pineapple**, **pony**.

How?

By giving the child opportunities to hear, and see, you say longer words that begin with **p** and to practise saying the words.

Resources

* Pictures of magnifying glasses (p. 149). Each magnifying glass has a hole in the lens. Cut out each magnifying glass and cut out the hole in each one.

* Large pictures of longer words that begin with **p** (pp. 150–161).

Instructions

1. Make sure the child cannot see the pictures, e.g. **paper** and **puddle**. Cover one of the pictures with the magnifying glass that has the smaller hole so that a bit of the picture can be seen through the hole.

2. Let the child have two or three guesses at what the picture is. If he cannot guess, change magnifying glasses so that the hole in the lens is bigger and more of the picture can be seen through it. Ask the child what he thinks the picture is.

Variation

* Put the doors (p. 59) on top of the page so that the pictures are covered. Take it in turns to open the doors and name the pictures.

Tips

*Help! The child says **pupple** instead of **puddle**! What can you do?*
* Break the word into two halves, e.g. **pu** and **ddle**. Leave a pause between the two halves: **pu** (pause) **ddle**. Gradually make the pause that you leave between the two halves of the word smaller until there is no pause and you are saying the word: **puddle**. Try some of the ideas described in the tips to help a child say longer words that start with **p** in Section 4, e.g. **park** (pp. 79–80). For example, put two paper hands

on the wall. Touch a hand and say **pu**. Touch the other hand and say **ddle**. Gradually bring the hands closer together, making the pause between **pu** and **ddle** smaller. When the child is ready, put the hands next to each other and say the word without a pause: **puddle**.

Help! The child still finds it hard to say longer words! He gets all the sounds muddled up! What can you do?

- It takes some children longer than others to say words. Children need to hear words many times in order to say the words correctly. They need lots of opportunities to practise saying the words you are working on, e.g. in activities and games. Regular repetition is important. Carry out work at the child's pace.

Finish my word (Speaking activity)

Aim
To say longer words that begin with the speech sound **p**, **pizza**, **pepper**, **poodle**, **puppy**, **poppy**, **paper**, **pillow**, **pebble**, **puddle**, **purple**, **popper**, **people**, **pasta**, **panda**, **pink**, **paint**, **pencil**, **parcel**, **pocket**, **pancake**, **peanut**, **pelican**, **pineapple**, **pony**.

How?
By giving the child opportunities to hear, and see, you say longer words that begin with **p** and to practise saying the words.

Resources
- Two sets of the small pictures of longer words that begin with **p** (pp.145–148)

Instructions
This activity is for children aged four and a half upwards.
1. Put at least three pictures in a line in front of the child, e.g. **panda**, **purple**, **paper**. Tell the child that you have a really bad memory and cannot remember the ends of words. Ask the child if he can help you name the pictures.

2. Say the first syllable of each word, e.g. "**Pan___**. Oh, what is it? **Pan ___**. I know it, I just can't quite remember it! **Pan___** "It's no good, I can't remember it! Can you help me?" See if the child can complete the word (**panda**). If he says '**da**', say the word aloud, "**Panda**! Of course! Thanks" and then ask him to say it for you, e.g. "Oh, no! I've forgotten it again! Can you help me again, please! What is it?"

Variations
- Put at least three pictures in front of the child. Ask him to listen carefully and point to the picture that you say, or put a counter on it, or hold it up. Break the word into syllables leaving a pause between the syllables, e.g. "**pur – ple**".

- Choose at least five pictures. Make sure the child has the same pictures that you have. Place a barrier between you and the child so that you cannot see each other's pictures. Say at least two words for the child, breaking the words into syllables, e.g. **pa – per**, **pan – da**. The child listens and arranges his pictures on his side of the barrier in the order he hears them. Ask the child what pictures he has so that he has to name them for you. Then remove the barrier to see if they match your pictures.

What did I say? (Listening and speaking activity)

Aim

To say longer words that begin with the speech sound **p**: **pizza**, **pepper**, **poodle**, puppy, **poppy**, **paper**, **pillow**, **pebble**, **puddle**, **purple**, **popper**, **people**, **pasta**, **panda**, **pink**, **paint**, pencil, **parcel**, **pocket**, **pancake**, **peanut**, **pelican**, **pineapple**, **pony**.

How?

By giving the child opportunities to hear, and see, you say longer words that begin with **p** and to practise saying the words.

Resources

At least two sets of the small pictures of longer words that begin with **p** (pp. 145–148).

Instructions

You are the speaker and the child is the listener in these activities.

1. Choose two pictures, e.g. **pizza** and **pebble**. Put them on the table in front of the child and name them for him: "**Pizza. Pebble**". Tell the child to listen carefully and then you name one of the pictures placed in front of him, e.g. "**Pebble**". Then say "What did I say?" The child listens and points to, or holds up, or puts a counter on the picture of the word he heard you say.

2. When you think the child is ready to listen and remember more words, choose three pictures, e.g. **poppy**, **pillow** and **pepper**. Put them on the table in front of the child and name them for him. "**Poppy. Pillow. Pepper**". Tell the child to listen carefully and then you name two of the pictures placed in front of him, e.g. "**Pepper. Pillow**". Then say "What did I say?" The child listens and points to, or holds up, or puts a counter on the words he heard you say. Increase the number of words to make the activity more challenging when you think the child is ready. For example, choose four pictures, name them, then name three of the four and ask the child to point to the three that you said.

Variations

To make the activity more challenging, present at least three pictures to the child. Write down the words in the order you are going to say them, not in the order they are in front of the child. For example, if the pictures in front of the child are **poppy**, **pillow**, **pepper**, you might write down **pepper**, **poppy**, **pillow**. Read out the words that you have written down: **pepper**, **poppy**, **pillow**. The child listens and arranges the pictures correspondingly, i.e. Pepper. Poppy. Pillow, to match what you said. To do this activity, the child needs to be able to write, but not spell!

Give the **same** pictures to yourself and to the child. You will need at least three, e.g. **panda**, **poodle**, **paper**. Place a barrier between yourself and the child so that you cannot see each other's pictures. Arrange your pictures without the child seeing. Name the pictures in the order you have arranged them, e.g. '**Paper. Panda. Poodle**'. The child listens and arranges his pictures to match what you have said. Remove the barrier and see if the child's pictures are in the same order as yours! **Reverse** the game so that the child is the **speaker** and you are the **listener**.

Tips

Help! The child can't remember what you said! What can you do?

- Start this activity by asking the child to remember one picture. Show him two pictures, e.g. **paper** and **poppy**, and name one of the pictures, e.g. **Poppy**. The child listens and points to the one that he heard. If he can do this easily, make the activity more challenging by presenting the child with three pictures, e.g. **pizza**, **puppy**, **pepper**, and naming two of them, e.g. '**Puppy. Pepper**'. Gradually increase the number of pictures so that the child has to remember more words. If he cannot remember what you said, try reducing the number of pictures you are using, e.g. use three pictures instead of four.

Help! The child can't write the words! What can you do?

- To take part in this activity, children have to be able to read what they have written to you, but this does not mean that they have to spell the words correctly. For example: they might write 'pupy' for 'puppy'. Ask an adult or another child to help.

- Draw pictures of the words that you are going to say to the child, instead of writing the words. The child can draw pictures of the words he is going to say in the activity. He might need some help from an adult or another child.

Help! It's really hard work to get the child to do these activities! What can you do?

- Make sure you don't do these activities for too long. If the child finds it hard to concentrate, keep them short and fun!

- Offer a reward to the child if he does, say, one activity. Choose a reward that you know he will enjoy, e.g. blowing bubbles, playing with Lego for five minutes. Gradually increase the number of activities he has to do in order to get the reward!

Roll and say (Speaking activity)

Aim

To say longer words that begin with the speech sound **p**, **pizza**, **pepper**, **poodle**, **puppy**, **poppy**, **paper**, **pillow**, **pebble**, **puddle**, **purple**, **popper**, **people**, **pasta**, **panda**, **pink**, **paint**, **pencil**, **parcel**, **pocket**, **pancake**, **peanut**, **pelican**, **pineapple**, **pony**.

How?

By giving the child opportunities to hear, and see, you say longer words that begin with **p** and to practise saying the words.

Resources

- One set of small pictures that have shapes on the back (pp. 145–148, 26).

- A dice.

- Template for a dice with a different shape on each face (p. 27).

Instructions

1. Spread the pictures out in front of the child, six at a time, face down so that you cannot see the pictures but you can see the shapes on the back.

2. Roll the dice with shapes on it. The shapes on the dice match the shapes on the back of the pictures. Turn over the picture that has the same shape as the dice, e.g. circle, so that you can see what the picture is, e.g. **poppy**.

3. Roll the dice with numbers on it. You have to say the word on your picture, e.g. **poppy**, the number of times that you throw on the dice, e.g. 5 "**poppy, poppy, poppy, poppy, poppy**". Make sure you have the first turn so that you can demonstrate the activity to the child.

Variation

- Make the game competitive: the winner is the first person to say the names of all of the six pictures in the activity, i.e. to throw all of the shapes on the dice.

- Roll the dice with shapes on it and turn over the picture that has the same shape on it, e.g. heart. Take it in turns to see how many times you can say the word in a minute. Use a one-minute salt timer.

My progress

Date	I can ...	☺/☹	I need to work on ...
	Listen carefully and hear long words that begin with **p**, e.g. **pillow**, **poodle**, **pizza**, without any help.		
	Listen carefully and hear long words that begin with **p**, e.g. **pillow**, **poodle**, **pizza**, with help.		
	Say **p** at the beginning of long words, e.g. **pillow**, **poodle**, **pizza**, without any help.		
	Say **p** at the beginning of long words, e.g. **pillow**, **poodle**, **pizza**, with some help.		

pebble

paper

pillow

puddle

pizza

pencil

pink

popper

parcel

puppy

pepper

poodle

pasta

pancake

poppy

people

peanut

pony

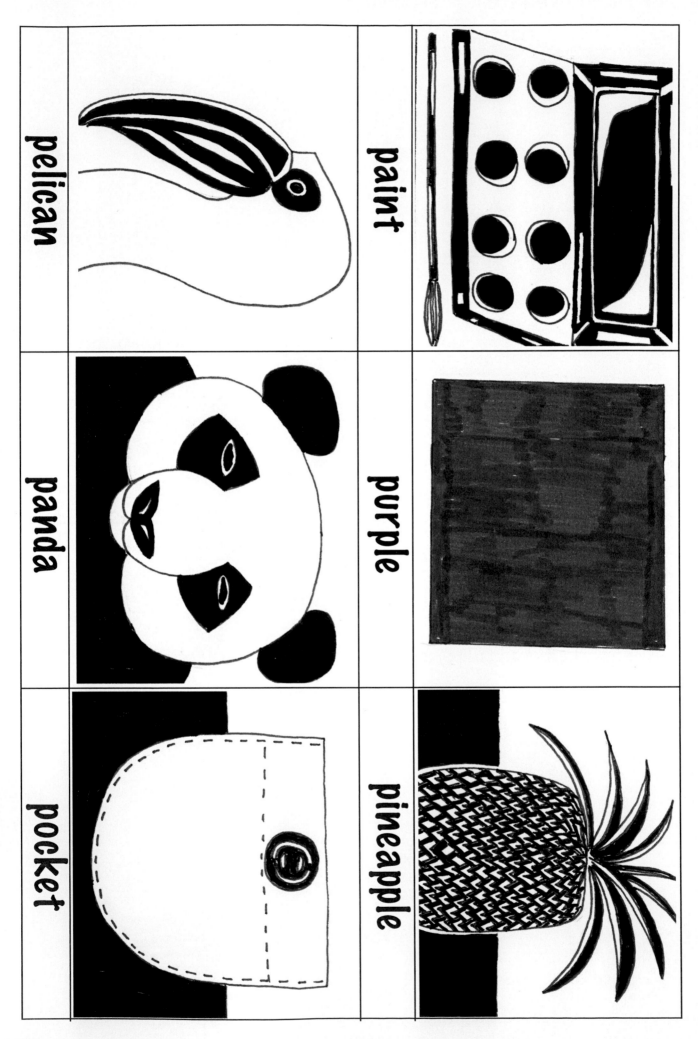

paint

purple

pineapple

pelican

panda

pocket

149

peanut

poppy

Look!

Look!

parcel

purple

pink

paint

Look!

Look!

pancake

people

pepper

poodle

Look!

Look!

pizza

pencil

155

popper

Look!

puppy

Look!

pasta

pony

pillow

pebble

Look!

puddle

paper

159

Look!

pelican

panda

Look!

pocket

pineapple

What's the next step?

- I can listen carefully and hear long words that begin with **p**, e.g. **pillow**, **poodle**, **pizza**, without any help. **Start working on Section 7. Continue playing listening games from the list of games in Section 8.**

- I can listen carefully and hear long words that begin with **p**, e.g. **pillow**, **poodle**, **pizza**, with help. **Continue doing listening activities from Section 6. Do listening activities from earlier sections to review work you have done with the child. Play listening games from the list of games in Section 8. When the child can hear long words that begin with p at least 70 per cent of the time in listening activities, start working on Section 7.**

- I can say **p** at the beginning of long words, e.g. **pillow**, **poodle**, **pizza**, without any help. **Start working on Section 7. Continue playing speaking games from the list of games in Section 8.**

- I can say **p** at the beginning of long words, e.g. **pillow**, **poodle**, **pizza**, with some help. **Continue doing speaking activities from Section 6. Do speaking activities from earlier sections to review work you have done with the child. Play speaking games from the list of games in Section 8. When the child can say long words that begin with p at least 70 per cent of the time in activities, start working on Section 7.**

Jingles with words that begin with p

See advice at the end of Section 3 on how to use the jingles in sessions (pp. 67–68)

Jingle one   (picture p. 166–167)

Listen

Pippa likes poodles
Paula likes ponies
Penny likes Pandas
Poppy likes cats!

Say the word

_____ (**Pippa**) likes poodles
_____ (**Paula**) likes ponies
_____ (**Penny**) likes pandas
_____ (**Poppy**) likes cats!

Jingle two (pictures p. 168)

Listen

Roly poly pudding and pie
What are we to do?
There's a puppy in a purple tie
And a pony in a shoe!

Say the word

Roly poly pudding and _____ (**pie**)
What are we to do?
There's a _____ (**puppy**) in a purple tie
And a _____ (**pony**) in a shoe!

Jingle three (pictures p. 169)

Listen

Dip, dap, doodle
I saw a poodle
Pip, pap, pee
The poodle saw me
Dip, dap, danda
I saw a panda
Pip, pap, pee
The panda saw me

Say the word

Dip, dap, doodle
I saw a _____ (**poodle**)
Pip, pap _____ (**pee**)
The _____ (**poodle**) saw me
Dip, dap, danda
I saw a panda
Pip, pap _____ (**pee**)
The _____ (**panda**) saw me

Jingle four
(pictures pp. 170–171)

Listen

A panda and a pony went across the sea
A panda and a pony ate a giant pea
A panda and a pony were chased by a giant bee
A panda and a pony were saved by me!

Say the word

A panda and a _____ (**pony**) went across the sea
A panda and a _____ (**pony**) ate a giant _____ (**pea**)
A _____ (**panda**) and a _____ (**pony**) were chased by a giant bee
A _____ (**panda**) and a _____ (**pony**) were saved by me!

Jingle five
(pictures pp. 172–173)

Listen

Can I have a pancake, please?
Can I have a pineapple pancake, please?
Can I have a pepper and pineapple pancake, please?
Can I have a pepperoni, pepper and pineapple pancake, please?
Yuk!

Say the word

Can I have a _____ (**pancake**), please?
Can I have a pineapple _____ (**pancake**), please?
Can I have a pepper and a _____ (**pineapple**) _____ (**pancake**), please?
Can I have a pepperoni, _____ (**pepper**) and _____ (**pineapple**) _____ (**pancake**), please?
Yuk!

Jingle six
(picture p.174)

Listen

Puppy, poppy, pippy
Pup, pop, pip
Paddle, puddle, piddle
Pad, pud, pid
Pebble, pubble, pibble
Peb, pub, pib
What a load of nonsense!

Say the word

Puppy, poppy, _____ (**pippy**)

Pup, pop, _____ (**pip**)

Paddle, puddle, _____ (**piddle**)

Pad, pud, _____ (**pid**)

Pebble, pubble, _____ (**pibble**)

Peb, pub, _____ (**pib**)

What a load of nonsense!

Look!

Pippa likes poodles

Paula likes ponies

Look!

Penny likes pandas

Poppy likes cats

Look!

A puppy in a purple tie!

A pony in a shoe

look!

a poodle

a panda

A panda and a pony

went across the sea!

ate a giant pea!

A panda and a pony

were saved by me!

were chased by a giant bee!

Can I have a

pancake, please?

pineapple pancake?

172

Can I have a

pepper and pineapple pancake?

pepperoni, pepper and pineapple pancake?

SECTION 7

SAYING P IN PHRASES AND SENTENCES

General advice

Choose which words you want to use in games. For example: you could start playing games using short words that begin with **p** (**pea**, **pear**, **pier**, **pow!**, **paw**, **pie**), then with longer words (**pot**, **pan**, **pig**, **pin**, **Paul**, **pipe**, **purse**, **peach**), and then with words with more than one syllable (**pizza**, **pepper**, **poodle**, **puppy**, **poppy**, **paper**, **pillow**, **pebble**, **puddle**, **purple**, **popper**, **people**, **pasta**, **panda**, **pink**, **paint**, **pencil**, **parcel**, **pocket**, **pancake**, **peanut**, **pelican**, **pineapple**, **pony**).

Try working with the same words until the child can say the words correctly in the games and activities most of the time, e.g. 70 per cent of the time. Then add some more words or change the set you are working on.

Try rotating sets of words. For example, work on up to ten words for a week and then work on a set of up to ten different words for another week, and another set of ten words for the third week; then go back to working on the first set of words.

Play games in small groups. This will increase the opportunities the child has to hear words with **p** and it will be fun!

Tell a story (Listening and speaking activity)

Aim
To say the words beginning and ending in **p** in phrases and sentences in games and activities.

How?
By giving the child opportunities to hear, and see, you say words in phrases and sentences and to practise the words.

Resources
- At least five small pictures, e.g. **pig**, **Paul**, **peach**, **pan**, **pin**.

- Computer or pen and paper to write a story, or a tape recorder or video recorder to record the child telling the story.

Instructions
1. Put the pictures face down in a pile in front of the child.

2. Turn over the first picture and make up the beginning of a story using the word, e.g. **Paul**. "Once upon a time there was a very tall boy called **Paul**."

3. Take it in turns to take a picture and make up the next part of the story using the word on it, e.g. **peach**. "**Paul** was hungry, but he didn't have any money to buy any food. He looked around to see what he could eat. Grass? No! Leaves? No! Then he saw a **peach**." Put the pictures face up on the table in a line as you use them in the story.

4. When you have finished the story, use the pictures to help the child remember and retell the story. Write the story on a computer or on paper or record it.

Make up sentences (Listening and speaking activity)

Aim

To say the words beginning and ending in **p** in phrases and sentences in games and activities.

How?

By giving the child opportunities to hear, and see, you say words in phrases and sentences and to practise the words.

Resources

- At least six small pictures, e.g. **pig**, **Paul**, **peach**, **pan**, **pin**,
- Paper and crayons, felt tip pens or coloured pencils.

Instructions

1. Put the pictures face down in a pile in front of the child.

2. Take it in turns to take a picture, e.g. **peach**, put the word in a phrase, e.g. 'a big, juicy **peach**', or in a sentence, e.g. 'I love **peaches**'.

3. Take it in turns to turn over two pictures, e.g. **Paul** and **pig**, and put both words in a phrase, e.g. '**Paul's** big **pig**', or a sentence, e.g. 'My friend **Paul** has a **pet pig**'.

4. Increase the number of pictures so that you increase the number of words that you have to put into a phrase or sentence, e.g. '**Paul's pig** likes to eat a **peach** in a **pot**'. See who can make the longest sentence!

5. See how many the child can remember.

Variations

- Write the phrases or sentences and illustrate them. Cover up the writing so that the child can only see the illustration. See if she can remember the phrase or sentence.

- Choose at least four words and make up a short rhyme or poem using the words.

- Take it in turns to throw a dice to see how many words you have to use in a sentence, e.g. 5, and make a sentence containing that many words, e.g. 'A **poodle** and a **pelican** fell in a **puddle** and a **pig** rescued them with a **paddle**.'

- See how many words that start or end with **p** the child can use in a sentence in one minute. Use a one-minute salt timer.

Make a word web (Listening and speaking activity)

Aim
To say the words beginning and ending in **p** in phrases and sentences in games and activities.

How?
By giving the child opportunities to hear, and see, you say **p** words in phrases and sentences and to practise the words.

Resources
- At least four small pictures, e.g. **poodle**, **pillow**, **pizza**, **pelican**.
- Paper, or a work book, or a photocopy of the blank template for a word web.
- Pencils, crayons or felt tip pens.

Instructions
1. Let the child choose one of the small pictures. Draw a circle in the middle of the piece of paper and write the word in it, e.g. **poodle**. Ask the child to draw it so you have a picture and the word.

2. Ask the child questions about the word. 'What is a **poodle**?'; e.g. a dog, an animal, a pet. 'Where does it live?' 'Where do you find it?'; e.g. in a house, in a kennel, in the park. 'What does it look like?'; e.g. it has four legs, a short tail, curly fur. 'What does it do?'; e.g. walk, run, eat, drink, sleep. 'Can you think of another dog/animal/pet?' 'Have you got a dog?'

3. Make a word web by drawing lines radiating out from the circle containing the word the child has chosen. Write the child's answers at the end of each line you have drawn, or in a shape at the end of each line, e.g. square, circle, triangle, or along each line. For example: 1. It is an animal. 2. You find it in the park. 3. It likes going for walks.

4. Keep the word webs in a work book or a word bag or folder. When you have at least three word webs, choose one. Make sure the child cannot see it. Tell the child about the word and ask them to guess what it is, e.g. 'It's an animal. It lives with people and it likes going for walks. What is it?'

5. Reverse this activity with older children so that they choose a picture and give you clues to guess what it is.

Board game variation (Speaking activity)

Aim
To say the words beginning and ending in **p** in phrases and sentences in games and activities.

How?
By giving the child opportunities to hear, and see, you say words in phrases and sentences and to practise the words.

Resources

- A board game, e.g. snakes and ladders.

- A set of the adjective cards, e.g. *big, hot, shiny (p.184)*.

- At least six small pictures of words you have been working on.

- A set of the emotions cards, e.g. *Say it in a happy voice, Say it in a sad voice, Say it in an angry voice (p.185)*.

Instructions

1. Set up the board game. Put the adjectives and the small pictures face down in two piles.

2. Take it in turns to take a card from each pile before you have your go, e.g. *hot*, **panda**.

3. Make a sentence using the two words, e.g. 'The **panda** was very *hot*.' Then have your go.

Variations

- Set up a board game and put a pile of the emotion cards and a pile of the small pictures face down. Before each go, players take an emotion, e.g. *angry*, and a small picture, e.g. **poodle**, and say the word in the manner of the adjective.

- Put a pile of the emotion cards and a pile of the small pictures face down. Take it in turns to take a card from each pile, e.g. *Say it in a tired voice* and **pie**, and say the word in the manner of the adjective. The other player has to guess what the adjective is.

- Put a pile of the emotion cards and a pile of the small pictures face down. Take it in turns to take a card from each pile, e.g. *Say it in a sad voice* and **poppy**. Make a phrase or sentence using the word, e.g. 'Pick a **poppy**', and say it in the emotion you have taken. See if the other player can guess what the emotion is.

Continue the sentence (Listening and speaking activity)

Aim

To say the words beginning and ending in **p** in phrases and sentences in games and activities.

How?

By giving the child opportunities to hear, and see, you say words in phrases and sentences and to practise the words.

Resources

- At least four small pictures, e.g. **poodle**, **pillow**, **pizza**, **pelican**.

Instructions

1. Put the small pictures face down in a pile.

2. You start by saying 'I went to the market and I bought a ...', and then take a picture from the pile, e.g. **puppy**.

3. The child says 'I went to the market and I bought a **puppy** and a ...' and then takes a picture from the pile, e.g. **pear**.

4. Keep going until a player cannot remember all the items they bought.

Variations

- Leave the pictures face up to help players remember what they bought.

- Change the place, e.g. 'I went to Jamaica and I saw ...'; 'I went to the moon and I took ...'.

Say the missing word (Listening and speaking activity)

Aim

To say the words beginning and ending in **p** in phrases and sentences in games and activities.

How?

By giving the child opportunities to hear, and see, you say words in phrases and sentences and to practise the words.

Resources

- At least one of the jingles that use the words you have been working on, e.g. 'Would you like **pea pie** or **pear pie**?'

Instructions

1. Read the jingle to the child at the end of a few sessions so that she knows it well.

2. Read the jingle, but do not say the last word of each line, e.g. 'Would you like pea pie or pear _____ (**pie**)?' and see if the child can remember the word and complete the sentence.

3. Gradually leave out more words in the jingle and see if the child can remember them, e.g. 'Would you like _____ (**pea**) pie or _____ (**pear**) pie?

Variations

- If the child cannot remember the words you have omitted from jingles, sound them out, e.g. **p – ie**. The child listens, puts the speech sounds together to make the word and says it, e.g. **pie**.

- Older children might be able to read some of the jingles with you.

Think of a word (Speaking activity)

Aim
To say the words beginning and ending in **p** in phrases and sentences in games and activities.

How?
By giving the child opportunities to hear, and see, you say words in phrases and sentences and to practise the words.

Resources
- Photocopy of the grid template *Can you think of ...?* and pencils or pens.

Instructions
1. Read the first question on the handout with the child, e.g. '*Can you think of an animal that begins with **p**?*'

2. The child has to think of a word that begins with **p**, e.g. **poodle, puppy, panda**. Write his answer on the handout and ask the second question, e.g. '*Can you think of a food that begins with **p**?*' Let the child look at the small pictures to help him think of answers if he needs support.

3. If the child can answer all the questions you could add further questions or the child could ask you further questions of his own!

Variation
- Make the activity into a competition. Players write their answers and do not show each other what they have written until the end.

Would you rather ...? (Listening and speaking activity)

Aim
To say the words beginning and ending in **p** in phrases and sentences in games and activities.

How?
By giving the child opportunities to hear, and see, you say words in phrases and sentences and to practise the words.

Resources
- The *Would you rather ...?* sheet. Cut it up and put the pieces in a pile face down.

Instructions
1. Take the first card from the pile. Read it out loud, e.g. '*Would you rather have a pot full of sweets or a pot full of money?*'

2. When the child answers the question, e.g. 'A pot full of sweets', ask her *Why?*

3. When the child has answered the questions, take another card and answer it.

4. Take it in turns to answer the *Would you rather ...?* questions.

Variations

- Make your own *Would you rather ...?* questions using words with **p** that you have worked on in this book.

- Older children might be able to read some of the *Would you rather ...?* questions.

- Carry out a survey with older children, e.g. ask teachers and children at least four of the *Would you rather ...?* questions and present the results.

I like / don't like ... (Listening and speaking activity)

Aim

To say the words beginning and ending in **p** in phrases and sentences in games and activities.

How?

By giving the child opportunities to hear, and see, you say words in phrases and sentences and to practise the words.

Resources

- The large *I like* and *I don't like* resource and the *I like / don't like ...* sheet giving different activities. Cut the sheet of paper up into cards and put the cards in a pile face down.

Instructions

1. Take the first card from the pile. Read the first part out loud, e.g. *playing in the* **park**.

2. Put the card on the 'I like' square or on the 'I don't like' square, depending on whether you like playing in the park or not. For example: 'I like playing in the park'.

3. Tell the child at least one thing about playing in the park, e.g. 'I like going on the swings. I like swinging as high as I can.'

4. Take it in turns to take a card, tell each other if you like it or not and tell each other one thing about it (see the cards for suggestions).

Variations

- Make your own versions using words with **p** that you have worked on in this book.

Adjectives

hot	cold	dirty
wet	big	small
long	short	hungry
thirsty	round	red
heavy	tall	shiny

Emotions cards

Say it in a tired voice	Say it in a happy voice	Say it in a sad voice
Say it in a loud voice	Say it in a quiet voice	Say it in an angry voice
Say it in a surprised voice	Say it in an excited voice	Say it in a scared voice
Say it in a low voice	Say it in a high voice	Say it in a bored voice

Can you think of …

an animal that begins with p?	
a colour that begins with p?	
a food that begins with p?	
a job that begins with p?	
a country that begins with p?	
a piece of clothing that begins with p?	
a sport that begins with p?	
a part of the body that begins with p?	
a name that begins with p?	

Would you rather ...

Would you rather eat pea ice cream or pea cake? Why?	Would you rather shake a lion's paw or a crocodile's paw? Why?
Would you rather dance with a pig or play football with a pig? Why?	Would you rather have a pot full of sweets or a pot full of money? Why?
Would you rather play with a panda in the park or with a pony? Why?	Would you rather hop to school or jump to school? Why?
Would you rather ride a sheep or ride a pig? Why?	Would you rather paint your bedroom pink or purple? Why?
Would you rather eat pasta or pizza? Why?	Would you rather stroke a panda or fly with a pelican? Why?
Would you rather take a pill to make you taller or take a pill to make you stronger? Why?	Would you rather take a ship to a desert island or take a ship to the North Pole? Why?
Would you rather walk a puppy or walk a poodle? Why?	Would you rather find a treasure map or a purse full of gold? Why?

I like	I don't like

I like / I don't like

eating peas + tell me one thing, eg another vegetable you like	eating pineapple + tell me one thing, e.g. your favourite fruit
eating pears + tell me one thing, e.g. another fruit you don't like	eating pizza + tell me one thing, e.g. your dream pizza
eating pasta + tell me one thing, e.g. your favourite pasta	jumping in puddles+ tell me one thing, e.g. when you last jumped in a puddle
wearing a cap + tell me one thing, e.g. what colour your baseball cap is	walking a puppy + tell me one thing, e.g. if you have got a puppy
playing in the park + tell me one thing, e.g. what you like playing on in the park	making pancakes + tell me one thing, e.g. what filling you put in your pancakes
painting pictures + tell me one thing, e.g. how often you paint	going on a ship + tell me one thing, e.g. where you have been on a ship, where would you like to go
wearing purple clothes + tell me one thing, e.g. what purple clothes you have got	poodles + tell me one thing, e.g. what your favourite dog is

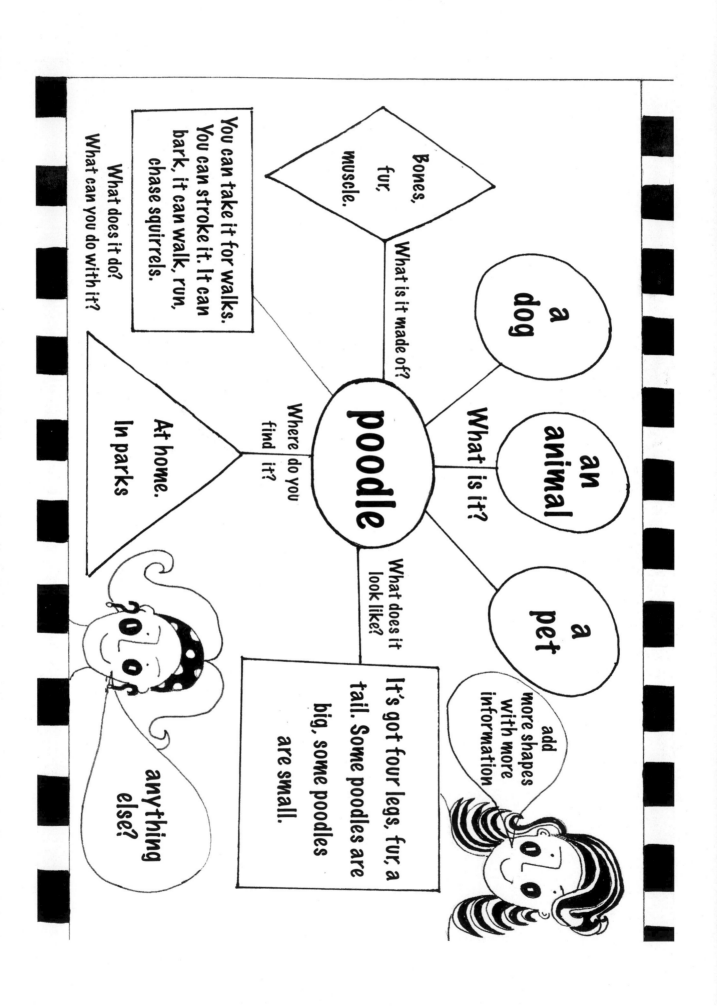

poodle

What is it?
- a dog
- an animal
- a pet

What is it made of?
Bones, fur, muscle.

What can you do with it?
What does it do?
You can take it for walks. You can stroke it. It can bark, it can walk, run, chase squirrels.

Where do you find it?
At home. In parks

What does it look like?
It's got four legs, fur, a tail. Some poodles are big, some poodles are small.

add more shapes with more information

anything else?

SECTION 8

GAMES TO PLAY WITH THE PICTURES OF WORDS BEGINNING AND ENDING WITH THE SPEECH SOUND P

Many of these games are suitable for paying with groups of children.

Contents

1. Pairs

2. Kim's game

3. Find the picture

4. Find the coin

5.   Which picture?

6. Catch a picture

7. Bowling

8. Goal!

9. What is it?

10. Draw it!

11. Guess what?

12. Listen and colour

13. Listen and do

14. Charades

15. Make a sentence (noughts and crosses)

Game 1: Pairs (Speaking game)

What you need to play
- At least two sets of small pictures of words you have been working on.

How to play
1. Shuffle the pictures and place them face down on the table.

2. Take it in turns to turn over two pictures.

3. Name each picture as you turn it over, e.g. "**Pan. Pin**".

4. If the pictures are the same, e.g. **park** and **park**, you keep the pair. If they are different, e.g. **pan** and **pin**, you put them back on the table face down. The winner is the person who has the most pairs of pictures.

Game 2: Kim's game (Speaking game)

What you need to play
- At least one set of the small pictures of words you have been working on.

How to play
1. Put at least three pictures in front of the child.

2. Name the pictures and talk about them with the child to make the pictures more memorable, e.g. "**Park**. I love going to the **park**. There is a **park** near my house. It's got a big climbing frame, swings, a slide and a roundabout. Do you like going to the **park**?" "**Pin**. Mind your fingers! It's sharp! Ow!"

3. Tell the child to look at the pictures and "take a photo" in his mind (mime taking a photo with an imaginary camera) to help him remember them.

4. Ask the child to close his eyes.

5. Take away one of the pictures.

6. Ask the child to open his eyes and see if he can remember what the missing picture is.

Variation
- Make the game more challenging by increasing the number of pictures you use and the number of pictures you take away when the child closes his eyes.

Game 3: Find the picture (Listening and speaking game)

What you need to play
- A set of the small pictures of words you have been working on.

- Some Blu-tack to stick the pictures around the room, e.g. on the door, on the back of a chair.

How to play
1. Show the child at least two pictures.

2. Name the pictures, e.g. "Look! **Pan** and **pig**". Talk about them a little to help the child remember the pictures.

3. Ask the child to close her eyes.

4. Hide the pictures and ask the child to open her eyes.

5. Ask her to find one of the pictures, e.g. "Find **pan**".

6. Reverse the game so that the child hides the pictures and tells you which one to find.

Variation
- Make the game more challenging by increasing the number of pictures you hide and the number of pictures you ask the child to find. For example: hide four pictures and ask the child to find two of them.

Game 4: Find the coin (Listening and speaking game)

What you need to play
A set of at least six small pictures of words you have been working on; a coin.

How to play
1. Put at least six of the small pictures in front of the child.

2. Name the pictures with the child, e.g. "**Park. Pill. Pin. Pot. Pan. Purse**".

3. Tell the child to close his eyes.

4. Hide the coin under one of the pictures.

5. Tell the child to open his eyes. The aim of the game is to find the coin. The child has to say which picture he thinks the coin is under, e.g. **pill**. Keep a record of how many guesses the child has before he finds the coin.

6. Reverse the game so that the child hides the coin and you guess which picture it is under. The winner is the person who finds the coin with the least number of guesses.

Variation

- Make the game more challenging by increasing the number of coins you hide. For example: hide three coins and the child has to guess which pictures they are under.

Game 5: Which picture? (Listening and speaking game)

What you need to play

- A set of small pictures of words you have been working on.

- Two cups (make sure you can't see through them).

- A coin or a counter or a small toy that will fit under the cups.

How to play

1. Choose two pictures and name them with the child, e.g. "**Pot. Pig**".

2. Turn the cups upside down and place them at the top of the pictures.

3. Tell the child to close her eyes and put the coin/counter/small toy under one of the cups.

4. Ask the child to open her eyes. The aim of the game is for the child to guess which cup the coin/counter/small toy is under. The child names the picture that the cup is on, e.g. "Pig" and then looks under the cup to see if the item is underneath.

5. Reverse the game so that the child hides the coin/counter/small toy and you guess which cup it is under.

Game 6: Catch a picture (Listening and speaking game)

What you need to play

- A set of small pictures of words you have been working on.

- Paper clips to attach to the pictures that you are using in the game.

- A fishing rod. Make a fishing rod by attaching some string to a piece of wood or a pencil and tie a small magnet to the end of the string.

How to play

1. Put a paper clip on each of the small pictures that you are using in the game. Place the pictures face down, so that you can't see them, on a flat surface or in a large bowl or similar container.

2. Take turns to "catch a fish" with the rod and name the picture, e.g. "**park**".

Variations

- See if you can catch a pair of pictures, e.g. **pea** and **pea**.

- Make sure the pictures are showing and take it in turns to tell each other what picture to catch: "Catch **pear**", "Catch **pie** and **pow**!" Make this game more challenging by increasing the number of pictures you ask each other to catch.

Game 7: Bowling (Listening and speaking game)

What you need to play
- A set of small pictures of words you have been working on.
- Two plastic bottles or skittles.
- Blu-Tack to stick the pictures on to the bottles or skittles.
- A small ball.

How to play
1. Choose two pictures, e.g. **purse** and **peach**.

2. Attach the pictures on to bottles/skittles with blue tak, e.g. put purse on one skittle and put **peach** on the other skittle, or put a picture under each skittle.

3. To play this game as a listening game, give the ball to the child. Name one of the pictures on one of the skittles, e.g. "**Purse**". The child listens and points to the picture that she heard you name. If she is right, she tries to knock the skittle over with the ball.

4. To play this game as a speaking game, let the child name one of the pictures, e.g. "Peach". You listen and point to the picture that you heard her name. If you are right, you roll the ball and try to knock over the skittle.

Game 8: Goal! (Listening and speaking game)

What you need to play
- A set of small pictures of words you have been working on.
- A bean bag or a small ball.
- Two boxes or containers, e.g. buckets
- Blu-Tack to stick the pictures on to the boxes or containers.

How to play
1. Choose two pictures of words that you have been working on, e.g. **purse** and **peach** Attach the pictures to the containers or place them in front of the containers.

2. To play this game as a listening game, give the beanbag/ball to the child. Name one of the pictures, e.g. "**Peach**". The child listens and points to the picture that he heard

you name. If he is right, he tries to throw the beanbag/ball into the appropriate container.

3. To play this game as a speaking game, let the child name one of the pictures, e.g. "**Purse**". You listen and point to the picture that you heard him name. If you are right, you throw the ball into the corresponding container.

Game 9: What is it? (Speaking game)

What you need to play

- At least one set of small pictures of words that you have been working on

- Plasticine or playdough.

How to play

1. Put the pictures face down in a pile in front of the players.

2. Take a picture from the pile. Do not show it to anyone else.

3. Take some playdough or Plasticine and make a model of the picture.

4. The child has to guess what it is.

5. Take it in turns to take a picture and make a model of it for the other player to guess what It Is.

Variations

- Limit the number of guesses to three!
- Give the child a minute to guess what your model is! Use a one-minute salt timer.

Game 10: Draw it! (Speaking game)

What you need to play

- At least one set of small pictures of words you have been working on

- paper and pencils or pens.

How to play

1. Put the pictures in a pile face down in front of the players.

2. Take a picture. Do not show it to anyone else.

3. Draw the picture.

4. Ask the child to guess what the picture is as you are drawing it.

5. Take it in turns to take a picture and draw it for the other player to guess what it is.

Variations

• Limit the number of guesses to six or fewer!

• Give the child a minute to guess what your picture is! Use a one-minute salt timer.

Game 11: Guess what? (Listening and speaking game)

What you need to play

• At least one set of small pictures of words you have been working on.

How to play

1. Choose a picture. Do not show it to anyone else.

2. Say three things about the picture for the child to guess what it is. For example: "It is a fruit. 'It is green'. It has pips. What is it?" (**pear**)

3. If this is too difficult for the child, put out at least three pictures and describe one of them. The child listens to your description and points to the picture.

4. Reverse the game where possible so that the child says three things about a picture and you guess what it is. If this is too hard, lower the number of clues to one or two. For example: Panda, "It's a black and white animal" (two clues).

Variations

• Limit the number of clues you give the child to four or fewer!

• Give the child a minute to guess what your picture is! Use a one-minute salt timer.

Game 12: Listen and colour (Listening and speaking game)

What you need to play

• Two identical sets of small pictures of words you have been working on, one for you and one for the child

• A barrier, that you can place between yourself and the child so that you cannot see each other's pictures.

How to play

1. With younger children, e.g. aged three to four, put at least two pictures in front of the child. e.g. park and pig.

2. Ask the child to colour one of the pictures, e.g. "Colour pig". To make the game more challenging increase the number of pictures and the number of colours, e.g. "Colour the **pig** red and the **pan** green" "Colour the **pig**'s legs blue and his nose orange".

Tip

Keep instructions short to make sure that the child can follow them. Children who are developing in a typical manner can usually follow instructions containing:

- two key words between the ages of 20 and 27 months, e.g. colour Pig's nose.

- three key words between the ages of 28 and 36 months, e.g. colour Pig's nose blue

- four key words between the ages of 34 and 42 months, e.g. colour Pig's nose and ears blue (Knowles 1982).

3. With children over four, make this game more challenging by placing a barrier between yourself and the child so that you cannot see each other's pictures. Put at least two pictures behind the barrier. Colour one of the pictures, or colour both of them using different colours. Then give instructions to the child, e.g. "Colour the **pig** green and the **pan** blue". When the child has finished, remove the barrier to see if you have coloured the same pictures.

4. Reverse the game where possible so that the child gives you instructions.

Game 13: Listen and do (Listening and speaking game)

What you need to play
- Two identical sets of small pictures of words you have been working on, one for you and one for the child.

- A selection of objects that are small enough to put on the pictures, e.g. a toy car, a button, a teaspoon, a toy animal, a small teddy. You need two of each so that you and the child have the same objects.

- A barrier that you can place between yourself and the child so that you cannot see each other's pictures.

How to play
1. Choose at least two pictures and two objects, e.g. **Paul** and **pot**, a car and a button. Put the objects on the pictures on your side of the barrier so that the child cannot see them. For example, put the car on the picture of Paul and the button on the picture of a pot.

2. Ask the child to do the same, e.g. "Put the car on **Paul** and the button on the **pot**". He listens to your instruction and arranges the pictures and objects on his side of the barrier.

3. When he has finished, raise the barrier to see if he has the same pictures and objects as you.

4. Reverse the game so that the child gives the instructions and you listen and do.

Game 14: Charades (Speaking game)

What you need to play
- A photocopy of the sheet with actions to perform, e.g. play in the park (opposite), cut up into separate actions.

How to play
1. Put the actions in a pile face down.

2. Take it in turns to pick up a card and mime what it says an action.

3. The winner is the person that guesses the most mimes correctly.

Variation
- Make up mimes with the child using the words you have been working on.

Charades

Pick a poppy!	Eat a juicy pear!
Make a pie!	Play in the park!
Mop the floor!	Eat some VERY hot soup!
Hop around the room!	Jump up and down!
Read the paper!	Throw a pebble in the sea!
Toss a pancake!	Turn the tap on and wash your hands!
Ride a pony!	Stroke a puppy!
Tread on a pin!	Put a tooth under your pillow!
Open a parcel!	Paint a picture!
Sail a ship!	Put some money in a purse!

Game 15: Make a sentence (noughts and crosses) (Speaking game)

What you need to play

- Pens or pencils, paper and at least nine words that you have been working on.

How to play

1. Draw a grid with nine boxes. Write one word in each box as in the examples below.

pear	peach	panda
pineapple	pot	Paul
pie	puppy	pancake

2. Take it in turns to choose a box. To put your nought or cross in the box, you have to make a sentence containing the word in the box. For example: "**Paul** is my best friend".

3. The winner is the person who gets a horizontal, vertical or diagonal line of noughts or crosses.

SECTION 9

SESSION PLANS

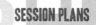

These session plans for a child aged 3 to 7, who is not saying the speech sound **p** in his talking. He may say **b** instead of **p**, for examples **bee** instead of **pea**, **bear** instead of **pear**.

Aim

To help him say **p** in his talking.

How?

- By showing him how his mouth works, e.g. tongue movements, lip movements.

- By helping him to hear the speech sound **p**, and to hear **p** at the beginning and end of words. The child might think he is saying **p**, so he thinks others can understand what he wants to tell them. You need to help him realise that he is not saying **p**, which can make it hard for others to understand what he wants to say.

- By helping him to make the speech sound **p** and then say **p** in words, e.g. **pie**, **pan**, **hop**.

1. To help the child to say the speech sound p – Section one and Section two.

What?	Why?	How?	Next step?
Mouth exercises	To help the child learn about her mouth and movements we make for speech.	**Section 1:** 1. Look in a mirror, e.g. "Show me your tongue. Show me your teeth activities". 2. Do single movements together with a mirror, e.g. "Can you put your tongue up to your nose".	**This is easy:** Sequence movements in Section 1, e.g. "Can you move your tongue up to your nose and down to your chin?" Play suggested games in Section 1 to practise sequences of mouth movements, e.g. roll a dice to get a number and do mouth movements that number of times.
Listening games	To help the child hear the speech sound **p**. To help the child hear that **p** and **b** are different speech sounds	**Section 2:** 1. Listening activities in Section 2, e.g. "Listen, when you hear me say p, put a pea on a plate" 2. Play listening games using **p** and **b** from the list of games in Section 8, e.g. Bowling (stick p on one skittle and b on the other), Catch a picture (fish for **p** and **b**), Listen and colour (colour **p** or **b**). 3. Play a listening game with the drawing activity in Section 2, e.g. "When I say **p**, colour in a ring".	**This is hard:** Keep working on single movements using a mirror. **This is easy:** Play the variation of this listening activity in Section 1 (listen to more speech sounds and put a pea on a plate when you hear **p**, e.g. **m, s, p, w, k**). Use more speech sounds in activities, e.g. put **b, p, s** on skittles. **This is hard:** Play the listening games with a toy/puppet so that the child can watch and listen. Play listening games with two sounds that are very different so that it is easier for the child to hear **p**, e.g. **p** and **s, p** and **k, p** and **w**.

What?	Why?	How?	Next step?
Speaking games	To help the child say the speech sound p.	**Section 2:** 1. Use a mirror so that the child can see your mouth and his mouth. Put a **pea** on **a** plate or a **pig** in the **pen** or **Paul** in the park and say **p**. Take turns to say **p** in this activity. 2. Use the drawing activities in Section 2 to practise saying p, e.g. "Say **p** and draw an eye on the alien". 3. Use **p** and other speech sounds in speaking games on the list of games in Section 8, e.g. Kim's game (present at least three speech sounds, e.g. **k**, **s**, **p**. The child closes his eyes and you take away one), Pairs, Which picture?	**This is easy:** Start working on words that begin with p in Section 3 (pea, pie, pear, pow! paw, pier) **This is hard:** 1. Do mouth movements to help the child learn about his mouth. 2. Play listening games so the child has lots of opportunities to hear p but does not feel any pressure to try to say p.

2. To help the child say p at the beginning of words – Section 1 and Section 3

What?	Why?	How?	Next step?
Mouth exercises	To help the child learn about his mouth and movements we make for speech.	**Section 1:** 1. Look in a mirror, e.g. "Show me your tongue. Show me your teeth." 2. Do single movements together with a mirror, e.g. "Can you put your tongue up to your nose/down to your chin?"	**This is easy:** Sequence movements in Section 1, e.g. "Can you move your tongue side to side?" Play suggested games in Section 1 to practise sequences of mouth movements, e.g. roll a dice to get a number and do mouth movements that number of times, e.g. 4. **This is hard:** Keep working on single movements using a mirror.
Listening games	To help the child hear **p** in words.	**Section 3:** 1. Listening activities in Section 3, e.g. present at least two pictures to the child, name one of them and the child holds up the one he heard you say. With children over four and a half years of age, play the listening games where you sound words out for the child, e.g. **p – ea (pea)**. 2. Play listening games from the list of games in Section 8 using the words in Section 3, e.g. Bowling, Catch a picture, Listen and colour. 3. Read the jingles from Section 3 to the child.	**This is easy:** Play listening games from Section 4. Play listening games with words that rhyme with the p words you are using, but start with b, e.g. **pea – bee, pier – beer, pear – bear, pie – bye**. For example: play Catch a picture, Listen and colour. **This is hard:** Play the listening games with a toy/puppet so that the child can watch and listen. Go back to playing listening games with p so that the child has more opportunities to hear the speech sound before you work on p in words.

What?	Why?	How?	Next step?
Speaking games	To help the child say the speech sound p in words.	**Section 3:** 1. Play speaking games from Section 3, e.g. open the door and name the picture, Hide the pea, Roll and say.. 2. Play speaking games from the list of games in Section 8 using the words from Section 3. 3. See tips at the end of Section 3 on using jingles as speaking activities, e.g. leaving a word out of a line of a jingle for the child to say.	**This is easy:** Start working on words that begin with p in Section 4, e.g. **park, pan, pipe.** **This is hard:** See tips in Section 3 for help. Go back to working on Section 2 and gradually introduce words and games from Section 3.

3. To help the child say p at the beginning of longer words – Section 1 and Section 4.

Tip: some children find it easier to say p at the end of words than at the beginning. If the child you are working with finds it easier to say p at the end of words, work on words from Section 5 before you work on words from Section 4.

What?	Why?	How?	Next step?
Mouth exercises	To help the child learn about her mouth and movements we make for speech. To warm up before starting work on saying **p** in words.	**Section 1:** Sequence mouth movements. Play mouth movement games from Section 1.	**This is easy:** Tell the child you are warming up before the hard work begins! Keep this section short and fun. **This is hard:** Keep working on single movements using a mirror.
Listening games	To help the child hear p in words.	**Section 4:** 1. Listening activities in Section 4, e.g. Listen and guess. With children over four and a half years of age, play the listening games where you sound words out for the child, e.g. **p – in (pin)**. 2. Play listening games from the list of games in Section 8 using the words in Section 4, e.g. Goal! 3. Read the jingles from Section 4 to the child. See tips on reading the jingles at the end of Section 3.	**This is easy:** Play listening games from Section 5. **This is hard:** Play the listening games with a toy/puppet so that the child can watch and listen. Go back to Section 3.

What?	Why?	How?	Next step?
Speaking games	To help the child say the speech sound p in words.	**Section 4:** 1. Play speaking games from Section 4, e.g. Roll and say, What's the word. 2. Play speaking games from the list of games in Section 8 using the words from Section 4, e.g. Guess what? 3. See tips on using jingles as speaking activities, e.g. leaving a word out of a line of a jingle for the child to say.	**This is easy:** Start working on words that end with **p** in Section 5, e.g. **mop**, **map**, **cup**. **This is hard:** See tips in Section 4 for help. Go back to working on Section 3 and gradually introduce words and games from Section 4.

4. To help the child say p at the end of words – Section 1 and Section 5

What?	Why?	How?	Next step?
Mouth exercises	To help the child learn about her mouth and movements we make for speech. To warm up before starting work on saying **p** in words.	**Section 1:** Sequence mouth movements. Play mouth movement games from Section 1.	**This is easy:** Tell the child you are warming up before the hard work begins! Like footballers and athletes do before a game or a race! Keep this section short and fun. **This is hard:** Keep working on single movements using a mirror.
Listening games	To help the child hear **p** in words.	**Section 5:** 1. Listening activities in Section 5, e.g. Listen and guess. With children over four and a half years of age, play the listening games where you sound words out for the child, e.g. **ma - p.** 2. Play listening games from the list of games in Section 8 using the words in Section 5, e.g. What is it? Catch a picture. 3. Read the rhymes from Section 5 to the child. See tips on reading the jingles at the end of Section 3.	**This is easy:** Play listening games from Section 6. Use the words from Section 5 and play listening games from earlier sections. **This is hard:** Play the listening games with a toy/puppet so that the child can watch and listen. Go back to Section 4 and gradually introduce words from Section 5.

What?	Why?	How?	Next step?
Speaking games	To help the child say the speech sound p in words.	**Section 5:** 1. Play speaking games from Section 5, e.g. Roll and say, What's the word?. 2. Play speaking games from the list of games in Section 8 using the words from Section 5, e.g. Kim's game. 3. See tips on using jingles as speaking activities at the end of Section 3, e.g. leaving a word out of a line of a jingle for the child to say.	**This is easy:** Start working on Section 6. **This is hard:** See tips in Section 5 for help. Go back to working on Section 4 and gradually introduce words and games from Section 5.

5. To help the child say p in words with more than one syllable – Section 1 and Section 6 (games from other sections using words from Section 6 optional)

What?	Why?	How?	Next step?
Mouth exercises	To help the child learn about his mouth and movements we make for speech. To warm up before starting work on saying p in words.	**Section 1:** Sequence mouth movements. Play mouth movement games from Section 1.	**This is easy:** Tell the child you are warming up before the hard work begins, like footballers and athletes do before a game or a race! Keep this section short and fun. **This is hard:** Keep working on single movements using a mirror.
Listening games	To help the child hear p in words.	**Section 6:** 1. Listening activities in Section 6, e.g. What did I say?. 2. Play listening games from the list of games in Section 8 using the words in Section 6. 3. Read the rhymes from Section 6 to the child. See tips on reading the jingles at the end of Section 3.	**This is easy:** Great! The child can hear the speech sound **p** at the beginning and end of words. **This is hard:** Play the listening games with a toy/puppet so the child can watch and listen. Go back to Section 5 and gradually introduce words from Section 6.

What?	Why?	How?	Next step?
Speaking games	To help the child say the speech sound p in words.	**Section 6:** 1. Play speaking games from Section 6, e.g. Finish my word. 2. Play speaking games from the list of games in Section 8 using the words from Section 6. 3. See tips on using jingles as speaking activities at the end of Section 3, e.g. leaving a word out of a line of a jingle for the child to say	**This is easy:** Start using words from the sections you have been working on in phrases or sentences in Section 7. **This is hard:** See tips in Section 6 for help. Go back to working on Section 5 and 4 and gradually introduce words and games from Section 6.

6. To help the child say p in words in phrases and sentences – Section 7.

What?	Why?	How?	Next step?
Using words that the child has worked on in the book in phrases and sentences in games and activities.	To help the child say the speech sound **p** in their talking.	**Section 7:** See the advice in Section 7 for using activities, e.g. how to choose words to work on. Play games little and often, e.g. play a game from Section 7 at least three times a week.	**This is easy:** Play games in groups, not just one to one with the child. Give activities to carers to play at home. **This is hard:** Play games one to one, keep playing games which are familiar for the child from the list of in Section 8 .

What next?

Make lists of words that contain **p**. Choose words that are useful for the child, for example names of family, friends, teachers, classmates, pets, towns, cities, television programmes, food. If you are working in a nursery or school, use topic or curriculum vocabulary if you can so that the child has more opportunities to hear these words and try to use them. For example, if the topic is: habitats, words could be damp, pollution, park, pond, etc.

Use five to ten words, depending on the child. Ask older children if there are any words that have **p** in them that they find difficult to say and would like to work on.

Make a list of the words and then make at least two copies of the words (so that you can play games like Pairs), laminate and cut them into word cards. Make a word box or word bag to keep the words in. Try to work on words at least twice a week for at least ten minutes each time. Follow the same procedure in each session.

Suggested sessions

- Take it in turns to take a word out of the bag/box. Say each word for the child, so that she can hear the word.

- Ask the child to say the word after you. Aim for the best production she can do. Help her if she finds it hard by breaking words into chunks (see tips on saying longer words and on saying **p** at the end of words for advice and examples). Try breaking words into syllables, e.g. **py – ra – mid**. Try starting at the end of the word, e.g. **mid, ramid, pyramid**. Keep this activity short.

Tips

- Ask the child to imagine saying the word before she tries to say it out loud.

- Ask the child to say the word to herself quietly at least three times and then say it out loud to you.

- Put a rhythm on longer words, e.g. tap them with your finger or nod your head as you say them, or do bigger movements, e.g. bend your knees on each syllable.

- Choose one or two activities or games from this book to practise saying words.

- When the child can say her words accurately at least 70 per cent of the time, add some more words. Keep a checklist of the words so that you can see progress.

- Review words regularly by taking a few out of the word bag/box and playing games and activities with them from this book.

- When the child is making good progress with the words, give her opportunities to use them in the nursery/classroom, e.g. using names that contain **p**, talking about the topic that the words are from.

- Have a one-minute challenge! The child talks about a topic of interest, or her weekend / holiday, etc. for a minute and she has to try really hard to say **p** accurately in words in the minute. Gradually increase the time to a two-minute challenge, a three-minute challenge. This is to help the child monitor her talking and correct errors, such as saying **b** instead of **p** in words.

References

Flynn L & Lancaster G (1996) *Children's Phonology Sourcebook*, Speechmark Publishing, Milton Keynes.

Knowles W (1982) *The Derbyshire Language Scheme*, Madoc Computers, Nottingham.

Grunwell P (1987) *Clinical Phonology*, 2nd edn, Croom Helm, London.

Holm A, Crosbie S & Dodd B (2005) 'Phonological approaches to intervention', Dodd B (ed), *Differential Diagnosis and Treatment of Children with Speech Disorder* (2nd edn), Whurr Publishers, London.

Ripley K, Daines B & Barrett J (1997) *Dyspraxia: a Guide for Teachers and Parents*, David Fulton Publishers, London.

Stackhouse J (1992) 'Promoting reading and spelling skills through speech therapy', Fletcher P & Hall D (eds) *Specific Speech and Language Disorders in Children*, Whurr Publishers, London.